HEALTH PROMOTION IN MIDWIFERY
PRINCIPLES AND PRACTICE

SECOND EDITION

Jan Bowden RGN, RM, FP cert, BSc(Hons), PGCEA, MSc
Lecturer in Midwifery and Women's Health,
Florence Nightingale School of Nursing and Midwifery,
King's College London, UK

Vicky Manning RGN, RM, MSc, PGCEA
Lecturer in Midwifery and Women's Health,
Florence Nightingale School of Nursing and Midwifery,
King's College London, UK

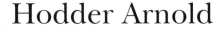
Hodder Arnold
A MEMBER OF THE HODDER HEADLINE GROUP

First published in Great Britain in 1997 by Arnold
This second edition published in 2006 by
Hodder Arnold, an imprint of Hodder Education and a member of the Hodder Headline Group,
338 Euston Road, London NW1 3BH

http://www.hoddereducation.com

Distributed in the United States of America by
Oxford University Press Inc.,
198 Madison Avenue, New York, NY10016
Oxford is a registered trademark of Oxford University Press

Whilst the advice and information in this book are believed to be true and accurate at the date of going to press, neither the
author[s] nor the publisher can accept any legal responsibility or liability for any errors or omissions that may be made.
In particular (but without limiting the generality of the preceding disclaimer) every effort has been made to check drug
dosages; however it is still possible that errors have been missed. Furthermore, dosage schedules are constantly being revised
and new side-effects recognized. For these reasons the reader is strongly urged to consult the drug companies' printed
instructions before administering any of the drugs recommended in this book.

British Library Cataloguing in Publication Data
A catalogue record for this book is available from the British Library

Library of Congress Cataloging-in-Publication Data
A catalog record for this book is available from the Library of Congress

ISBN-10   0 340 888 806
ISBN-13   978 0 340 888 803

1 2 3 4 5 6 7 8 9 10

Commissioning Editor: Clare Christian
Project Editor: Clare Patterson
Production Controller: Jane Lawrence
Cover Designer: Nichola Smith

Typeset in 10/12 Minion by Charon Tec Ltd, Chennai, India
www.charontec.com
Printed and bound in Malta.

What do you think about this book? Or any other Hodder Arnold title?
Please send your comments to www.hoddereducation.com

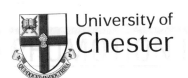
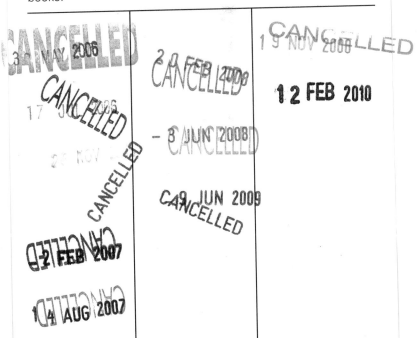

CONTENTS

CONTRIBUTORS

Gill Aston RGN, RM, ADM, PGCEA, MA, PhD
Lecturer in Midwifery and Women's Health,
Florence Nightingale School of Nursing and
Midwifery, King's College London, UK

Beverley Bogle RN, RM, MTD, Cert Counselling, Cert
Examining, Dip Nursing Part A, BEd(Hons), MSc, Family
Planning Cert, Cert Training for Trainers in Sexual Health
Lecturer in Midwifery and Women's Health,
Florence Nightingale School of Nursing and
Midwifery, King's College London, UK

Jan Bowden RGN, RM, FP Cert, BSc(Hons), PGCEA, MSc
Lecturer in Midwifery and Women's Health,
Florence Nightingale School of Nursing and
Midwifery, King's College London, UK

Penny Charles RGN, RM, DPSM PGCEA, BA(Hons),
MSc, Dip Aromatherapy
Lecturer in Midwifery and Women's Health,
Florence Nightingale School of Nursing and
Midwifery, King's College London, UK

Heather Finlay RGN, RM, BA(Hons), MSc,
PG Dip, PG Cert
Sure Start Midwife and Lecturer Practitioner
in Midwifery and Women's Health, Florence
Nightingale School of Nursing and
Midwifery, King's College London, UK

Moyra Heggie RGN, NDN, HV Cert, RM, Cert Family
Planning, MTD, BSc(Hons), MSc
Formerly Lecturer in Midwifery and
Women's Health, Florence Nightingale
School of Nursing and Midwifery, King's
College London, UK

Louise Long RGN, RM, BSc(Hons), PCGEA, MSc
Lecturer in Midwifery and Women's Health,
Florence Nightingale School of Nursing and
Midwifery, King's College London, UK

Vicky Manning RGN, RM, MSc, PGCEA
Lecturer in Midwifery and Women's Health,
Florence Nightingale School of Nursing and
Midwifery, King's College London, UK

Eddie West-Burnham BA, MSc
Sexual Health Co-ordinator, Cambridge
and Peterborough Public Health Network,
Huntingdon, UK

FOREWORD

I would like to start by saying how pleased I am that Health Promotion in Midwifery has reached a second edition, the first having been more popular than my editors at Arnold or I had ever dreamed possible. The development of the principles and practices laid out in this second edition will enable midwives and other health professionals to keep health promotion at the forefront of their midwifery practice. The popularity of this, and other publications, demonstrates that midwifery and health promotion are very comfortable partners in the minds and hearts of midwives.

While many of the principles of health promotion have followed a continuing pattern of growth and development in recent years, the popularity of the term 'public health' has re-entered British politics and health care, with an increasingly stronger emphasis being placed on preventative health care, social support of disadvantaged families and health protection that explores environmental threats to health. All of these require the input of midwives and midwifery to move our understanding of health issues forward, and no other health profession is so ideally placed to enable women and young families to benefit from increasing good-quality information that is fairly distributed and sensitively shared. This book will enable midwives to learn about many different aspects of health promotion, to consider how best to put that information into practice, and how we prepare future generations of mothers and midwives to gain improvements in the health of people and populations.

Although societies rely on Governments and Health Departments to lay down the parameters of how we approach public health and finance initiatives and care, it should never be forgotten that it is individual midwives who meet and influence individual women and their families, and can make real differences to how those people deal with health issues during their childbearing years and beyond. This book will help midwives to conduct their professional lives with greater understanding, deeper knowledge and better skills. It can be used to help midwives and student midwives to formulate questions and relate the principles and practice described to the reality of what they see, and how they work. Examples of some of the questions readers may wish to address are:

- What are the major health issues that need to be addressed in local midwifery practice (examples may be obesity in pregnancy, mental health issues, how parent education is delivered)?
- How are recent Government reports being interpreted locally to address health needs?
- Are my colleagues and I asking women the right questions at antenatal bookings, and subsequently? Are the right support mechanisms in place to follow up women with specific health needs, be they physical, psychological, social or environmental, or a combination of these?
- How are data on maternal and neonatal health outcomes being collected locally, and how are the results incorporated into practice, especially by midwives?
- What local research, audit and education are in progress, looking at and disseminating how the role of the midwife can best meet the health needs of the local population?

Midwives undoubtedly have an increasingly important role to play in improving the health of women and babies. It is an exciting time to be a midwife despite (or perhaps because of) the complexities and dilemmas which face us in practice every working day of our lives.

Helen Crafter
Senior Lecturer in Midwifery
Faculty of Health and Human Sciences
Thames Valley University
London, UK

PREFACE

Health promotion is very much part of the Government's agenda for reducing inequalities in health. Current Government policy and strategy clearly identify midwives as an integral part of their plans. Health promotion is not a new concept for midwifery and is a major part of what it is to be a midwife. Some may argue that almost everything a midwife does has an impact on, or link to, promoting the health of the woman, her fetus/baby and her family. As we discover more about the effect of the environment (*in utero* and generally), the ability to influence health in the short and long term is becoming more apparent. This includes environmental and social factors and, as a profession, midwifery is striving to face these issues and provide individualized care based on the needs of the woman.

The principles of general health promotion, such as models of care, good communication and information giving, and understanding basics of psychology, social and cultural issues, ethics and education, are important to the underpinning of good midwifery practice. This book attempts to bring together these concepts in a way that is user friendly and accessible, and encourages midwives to look at their wider public health role. However, midwives do not work alone, but with many allied professions in partnership, such as complementary therapy practitioners, primary health-care trusts and public health networks. Practice issues and frameworks related to providing health promotion within the multidisciplinary team are discussed and there are links and suggestions for further reading to lead on to the wider issues that we were unable to cover in this book.

Midwives today work in such diverse areas that each midwife, in their own way, needs to adapt their care to meet the needs of the woman, her family, the service and the Government's expectations. This book is intended to be realistic and practical in its suggestions for the promotion of health and for the provision of holistic care that is woman focused.

Jan Bowden and Vicky Manning

ACKNOWLEDGEMENTS

We would like to thank our families. Jan sends special thanks to her nan, sister Rae and niece Ellis for their ever-present love and support and Vicky sends special thanks to her husband who has been very supportive. We would also like to thank the following: our friends who have, in their own distinctive styles, found ways both big and small to encourage, support and advise us, read through drafts and provide much-needed light-heartedness and occasional solace via email, text, telephone and in person; Pauleene Hammett, our head of section, for being a brilliant, under-standing and caring friend as well as a boss; all the chapter writers for their professional expertise and knowledge – it has been a unique and rewarding experience to work with each of them; Sue Scullard and Terry Bowdery in the design department at King's College London Florence Nightingale School of Nursing and Midwifery, for making such clear diagrams out of vague ideas; Helen Crafter for setting a high standard in her original text and for providing the foreword for this second edition; and Clare Christian and Clare Patterson at Arnold for their much-needed help and advice.

Jan Bowden and Vicky Manning

Chapter 5
I would like to acknowledge Gill Aston's support during the writing of this chapter.

Jan Bowden

Chapter 8
I would like to thank Pauleene Hammett for her support and for allowing me to use the curriculum document that she authored.

Vicky Manning

Chapter 9
I would like to say a big thank you to my son Richard for all his support and help during the writing of this chapter.

Eddie West-Burnham

Chapter 10
I would like to thank those pre- and post-registration students who have, over many years, shared their thoughts, feelings and professional concerns regarding the sexual health-care needs of their clients. Acknowledgement of their increasing confidence and comfort in addressing their clients' sexual health concerns has been the inspiration for writing this chapter.

Beverley Bogle

Chapter 11
I would like to thank Nicki Adams for all her help with the structure.

Louise Long

Chapter 14
I would like to thank Dr Loraine Bacchus for her friendship and support in preparing the chapter on domestic violence.

Gill Aston

Chapter 15
I would like to thank my partner Jean-Luc and children Anäis and Luc for their good-hearted sharing of my time and focus for this chapter, and the editors Jan and Vicky for their good-natured help.

Penny Charles

LIST OF FIGURES

LIST OF TABLES

1 PUBLIC HEALTH, MIDWIFERY AND GOVERNMENT POLICY

HEATHER FINLAY

Public health is about enabling the population to live healthier lives. Definitions of what is meant by public health can be very broad, as this Government definition illustrates:

> *Public health [is] ... the science and art of preventing disease, prolonging life and promoting health through the organised efforts and informed choices of society, organisations, public and private, communities and individuals ...*
>
> *Wanless (2004, p. 3)*

Public health has been a part of Government policy from the days of the Victorian philanthropists' drive to end infectious diseases to the present Government's interest in healthy lifestyles. Different administrations have had both a different emphasis and a different commitment to public health.

Successive governments have for many years conveyed public health advice via health professionals. Midwives are no exception to this and from the turn of the nineteenth century part of the role of the midwife was to give both advice and instruction to women under their care (Leap and Hunter 1993). The midwife's role still includes giving what is essentially public health advice, to the woman, her partner and her family.

It could be argued that the current Government policy is an extension of this advice-giving role as the emphasis appears to be on targets around increasing breastfeeding rates and reducing the rates of smoking among pregnant women (Department of Health (DoH) 2004a). However, the reality is more complex because underpinning the Government policy is a desire to reduce health inequalities associated with disadvantage. It is this underlying public health initiative and the implications for both midwifery practice and service delivery that are considered in this chapter.

BACKGROUND TO MIDWIFERY, PUBLIC HEALTH AND GOVERNMENT POLICY

Midwifery care has always included a public health component, although the public health role is more apparent in community-based care (Henderson 2002). Provision of information around such topics as breastfeeding and women's health is recognizably part of the health promotion role of the midwife. However, midwifery connects with the broader definition of public health given at the start of this chapter. As a profession midwifery acknowledges childbirth as a psychological and social event rather than a purely clinical event and that optimum outcomes are the result of individual, community and organizational effort (Edwards et al. 2005). In essence midwives have understood that childbirth and raising a family are more than just a medical event and that the outcomes depend on the mother and the family's social and psychological circumstances as much as on the input of health professionals.

The contextual nature of childbirth has often been at odds with the organization of midwifery care within acute trusts. This has resulted in a tension between midwifery care in hospitals (which emphasizes acute interventions) and midwifery care that is community based (dealing with the larger public health agenda through giving care rooted in women and their families' everyday lives). This has led to much of the public health role of midwives beyond mere information and advice giving being tacit and unacknowledged (Henderson 2002).

It is against this background that Government policy has increasingly required midwives, and the NHS overall, to be more overtly involved in public health over the last 15 years. The *Health of the Nation* policy document (DoH 1992) acknowledged the need to promote health as well as to treat illness. This document has been criticized for its emphasis on the role of the individual in maintaining health while minimizing the role of external influences, but despite this it signalled a belief in the importance of public health. Since the Labour Government took office in 1997 there has been an increased recognition of the broader meaning of public health and an acceptance of the influence of disadvantage on health outcomes. The *Independent Inquiry into Inequalities in Health* (Acheson 1998) established a broad public health agenda that was followed through with *Saving Lives: Our healthier nation* (DoH 1999) and *Tackling Health Inequalities: A cross cutting review* (DoH 2002). The public health role of the midwife was specifically mentioned in *Making a Difference: Midwifery action plan* (DoH 2001). It is proposed that the postnatal contact with clients be lengthened to include the 6-week check. Both *Choosing Health: Making healthy choices easier* (DoH 2004a) and the *National Service Framework for Children, Young People and Maternity Services* (DoH 2004b; referred to in the text as the NSF) place midwifery care at the centre of the public health agenda. Both documents acknowledge that this placing of maternity care in a community context and actively engaging with disadvantaged communities can have positive consequences for the short- and long-term health of women and their children. This signals the beginning of an organized effort to promote health and prevent disease both within communities and with individuals, with a focus (certainly within the NSF) on preventing inequalities even before birth. Thus, midwifery can be seen as central to the execution of a broad concept of public health.

WHY NOW? FACTORS INFLUENCING GOVERNMENT OPINION ON MIDWIFERY AND PUBLIC HEALTH

The public health policy of the current Labour Government explicitly accepts the link between disadvantage, inequalities and health outcomes. The current thrust of public health policy is that disadvantage begins before birth and can be compounded after birth. So maternity care is fundamental to tackling the origins of disadvantage around the time of birth. The NSF sets a standard of increased equity of access to maternity services that it claims will:

> Increase the survival rates and life chances of children from disadvantaged backgrounds ...

DoH (2004b, p. 6)

The direction of Government policy comes as a response to increasing evidence of the short- and long-term consequences of disadvantage on maternal and child health. In fact the Government is measuring changes in health inequalities through tracking infant mortality (DoH 2004a). It has been known for some time that the outcomes for babies born to mothers who are disadvantaged are worse than for other groups. One example is the outcomes for children born to teenage mothers, where the infant mortality rate is 7.9:1000 live births. This mortality rate is almost twice that of infants born to the 30–34 year age groups (DoH 2004a). Teenage mothers are more likely than other age groups to be poor and have features of social exclusion (Palmer et al. 2004). Adverse outcomes for infants born to disadvantaged mothers are not just about mortality but are also reflected in long- and short-term morbidity. Much of the morbidity is as a result of the excess numbers of low-birthweight infants born to women in disadvantaged groups. Lone mothers are especially vulnerable and they can have almost twice the proportion of low-birthweight babies compared with women in stable relationships (Palmer et al. 2004). It is known that being born with a low-birthweight is associated with increased risk of death in the first year, disability and special educational needs (Royal College of Midwives (RCM) 2003).

The sixth report of the *Confidential Enquiry in Maternal and Child Health* (CEMACH) (Lewis and Drife 2004) has identified risk factors for maternal mortality that are no longer just medical. The risk factors identified by the sixth report are as follows (Lewis and Drife 2004, p. 26):

- Social disadvantage
- Poor communities
- Minority ethnic groups
- Late booking or poor attendance
- Obesity
- Domestic violence
- Suboptimal clinical care
- Lack of interprofessional or interagency communications.

The figures that emerge are stark; one example is that women from families where neither they nor their partners worked were 20 times more likely to die than women from more advantaged groups. Similarly, women who lived in the most deprived areas of the country had a 45 per cent higher death rate than women who lived in the most affluent areas. Women from black and minority ethnic groups also had poorer outcomes, with black African women having a mortality rate seven times that of the white population (Lewis and Drife 2004).

The CEMACH report (Lewis and Drife 2004) also recognizes the relationship between a woman and her family's psychosocial environment and health outcomes. The report identified key recommendations highlighting how the maternity services are failing to respond to the needs of the most vulnerable disadvantaged women in five crucial ways:

1. The current patterns of care are criticized for not being flexible enough to meet the needs of all women; the fact that many of the women who died found it difficult to access or maintain contact with the maternity services is commented on.
2. Many of the women who died were not followed up adequately when they failed to attend for care, despite having known risk factors.
3. The provision of multidisciplinary care was found to be patchy in part and it is suggested that both clinical and social service networks should be established for women with pre-existing medical, psychological or social problems.
4. The report recommends that women with complex needs should be offered appropriate care and the advocacy of a known midwife throughout their pregnancy.
5. An increased use of interpreters and a consideration of prejudices within the system are also recommended.

These five recommendations are more than just a reorganization of the maternity services. They are about public health and the role of the maternity services in preventing disease and prolonging life. The next section will consider how these recommendations have been translated into practice in *Choosing Health: Making healthy choices easier* (DoH 2004a) and the NSF.

CURRENT POLICY ON PUBLIC HEALTH

The current Government policy on midwifery and public health is encapsulated in two main documents.

Choosing Health (DoH 2004a)

This document is broader in scope than the NSF and looks generally at public health. Having said this, it contains ideas and strategies that echo the findings of the CEMACH report (Lewis and Drife 2004), plus some specific discussion of maternity services. Within this policy document it is highlighted that the current maternity services on offer are difficult to use and do not meet the needs of deprived groups and communities; in addition there is emphasis on the need for partnership working between services and between services and the communities that they serve. Tackling inequalities is also stressed as an integral component of improving public health. Midwifery is specifically mentioned as part of the support given to parents during pregnancy in order to break the cycle of inequalities between generations. The important role that midwives have in public health is recognized and there are five areas specifically mentioned:

1. Helping pregnant women stop smoking
2. Improving nutrition

3. Improving breastfeeding rates
4. Promoting mental health
5. Building social support.

National Service Framework for Children, Young People and Maternity Services (DoH 2004b)

This policy document is concerned with the care and treatment of children and young people in the health and education sectors and with maternity services. It offers 11 standards, which should provide a nationwide standard by identifying markers of good care. Standard 11 is specifically concerned with maternity services and brings together many of the themes that have already been noted in both the CEMACH report (Lewis and Drife 2004) and *Choosing Health* (DoH 2004a). The markers of good practice identified in the NSF begin with the idea of a proactive maternity service, acknowledging that disadvantaged groups with complex needs have the least access to services, a theme in both CEMACH (Lewis and Drife 2004) and *Choosing Health* (DoH 2004a). The NSF sets a standard that is about reaching out to women who are marginalized and at risk of poor outcomes:

> Maternity services are proactive in engaging all women, particularly women from disadvantaged groups and communities, early in their pregnancy and maintaining contact before and after birth.
>
> DoH (2004b, p. 5)

There is also confirmation within the NSF of the Government's objective to involve local communities in developing and planning services. The aim of this objective is to ensure that services are developed in partnership with the communities in such a way that they are a 'best fit' for the local community, especially the vulnerable women and families within that community (see Chapter 9). It is becoming increasing apparent that current maternity services are not meeting the needs of certain groups of women and their families. In theory the increased autonomy given to primary care trusts (PCTs) and foundation hospitals will provide the flexibility for services to be configured to provide the 'best fit' for local needs. The problem with this is how best to ensure that the local community is involved in developing local services.

Historically, maternity services have had input from local communities through the maternity services liaison committees (MSLCs). In practice many MSLCs have been disbanded partly as a result of a lack of incentives to attend and difficulty in ensuring that they are representative of the local community, especially in terms of groups with more complex needs (RCM 2003). The NSF acknowledges the link between uptake of services and local women and families being involved in the planning of services. This is a bold statement. Meaningful engagement with the local community in the planning of services will be a challenge to the power of the service providers. It could even be a challenge to midwives because local communities may decide that they do not like or want the services that the professionals feel should be provided for them. So, the success of community involvement may depend on the willingness of the service providers to allow local communities ownership of health projects and to give the local community the ability to make real changes to the care provided.

A possible model for enhancing community involvement could come from the Sure-Start initiative where local boards are made up of local parents (who are elected at annual general meetings) and local service providers. One of the features of some Sure-Start schemes has been a willingness to get out into the community to find and recruit local women, e.g. going to local play groups, and talking to women at school gates and at doctors' surgeries. Board meetings are locally based, child care is provided and travel costs are reimbursed where necessary. In addition, the Sure-Start boards have the power to decide the direction of the local Sure-Start scheme and its budgets. It will be interesting to see how the enhanced community involvement envisaged in the NSF evolves in reality.

Specific services are also mentioned in the NSF for women, and their partners where applicable, who are requesting help and support with domestic violence, stopping smoking, substance misuse and mental health problems. The groups identified are almost identical to the main classifications of women who, alongside disadvantaged women, are deemed to be 'at risk' by the CEMACH report (Lewis and Drife 2004).

Helping pregnant women to stop smoking, encouraging good nutrition (particularly through the healthy start welfare food scheme) and increasing breastfeeding rates are also mentioned in the NSF. An improvement in these areas is linked to the Government's overall standards for improving public health, although there are specific benefits for pregnant women and their babies. The benefits for women and children are better rates of mortality and morbidity, plus better life chances.

IMPLEMENTING PUBLIC HEALTH: WHAT MIGHT IT MEAN?

The implementation of the NSF will be a major challenge. The extent to which its vision is realized will depend on the ability of local trusts to introduce the changes in service provision and focus outlined in the NSF, which include organizational change, the focus of maternity care and multidisciplinary working.

Organizational change

The NSF identifies three areas of possible organizational change.

Community focus

The NSF promotes a change in the organization of maternity care so that services are actively designed to overcome barriers to care. This is part of the move towards a proactive service that reaches out to vulnerable women. This will require a change in the configuration of the service as well as a change in midwifery attitudes and values to ensure that public health is given a comparable status to other parts of the service. As pointed out earlier the women with the worst maternal and neonatal outcomes are often those who do not use or under-use the maternity services. As a response to this the NSF proposes an expansion of community-based care. One of the suggestions is having midwives based at children's centres where they will be visible and accessible, plus two visits by a midwife early in pregnancy so that a woman can discuss her care. An expansion of community-based care has the potential to help women access services early, e.g. having midwives in the children's centre at the same time as free pregnancy testing at a family planning clinic, both in the same venue, plus midwives who spend most of their time in the community may be in a better position to follow up women who do not attend for antenatal care.

Flexibility of service provision

The NSF notes that maternity services may be provided in places and at times that make it difficult for women to access the services. It suggests that services should be re-designed, taking into account the reasons why disadvantaged women have found it difficult to access care. This suggests a more fundamental change than just expanding current community care, because community care obviously has not protected vulnerable women in its current form. So, perhaps more flexibility within service provision needs to be considered. Maternity services could be based around women and their families' needs rather than women and their families having to adapt to the service's needs if they want access to care.

There are many examples of flexible care, largely given in women's homes, which may provide a model for service change (Greenwood 2004). Sure-Start schemes have also given examples of how to help women engage with services; an example is using local community volunteers (who are then rewarded for their time) to accompany women to services or groups when women are unsure of going alone. The concept of flexibility in service provision suggested in the NSF extends beyond merely organizational change and has implications for clinical care, especially postnatal care. The NSF (DoH 2004b, p. 34) advocates that women be discharged from the maternity service 'according to their individual needs and those of their babies'. The routine 10- to 14-day discharge still seems to miss many post-delivery health problems and it is too short for midwives to ensure that the necessary support mechanisms are in place for women with complex physical, psychological or social needs. The NSF suggests that the time women and their families receive care from the midwifery-led services should be at least a month and up to 3 months, depending on individual need. This is a major change in service provision and has obvious resource implications. However, the NSF discusses the integration of maternity support workers, peer support initiatives and Sure-Start early years' services as part of the package of care during the extended period.

Continuity of care

As part of a maternity service that is community focused and flexible, the NSF envisages midwives being easily contactable day or night and accessible for all women in a community. In addition all women should have the support of a named midwife throughout pregnancy. It could be argued that at present all women can contact a midwife by phone at a hospital, on either a labour ward or a delivery suite 24 hours a day. However, little is known about the quality of the interaction in a situation where the midwife may not know the woman calling. Where midwifery services are working with women from disadvantaged and minority groups and communities it is proposed by the NSF (DoH 2004b, p. 14) that 'community-based continuity of care schemes' be developed. This is in line with the CEMACH report (Lewis and Drife 2004), which recommends that women with complex pregnancies receive the support and advocacy of a known midwife throughout the pregnancy. The role of the midwife in this situation is to act as a support and advocate for the woman while giving midwifery care, in addition to any specialist care that the woman is receiving. In addition, the knowledge that the midwife has of the woman and her care means that the midwife can ensure that care does not falter, either through a problem with the service providers or through the woman being unable to attend appointments.

The focus of maternity care

The official focus of maternity care for the last 100 years has been medical. At its most basic the provision of maternity care has been to keep mothers and their babies alive and well. There has been a huge improvement in outcomes for women and their babies and these improvements have been a direct result of advances in medical and midwifery care. However, there has been a growing realization that to reduce maternal mortality further the maternity services have to be aware of the relationship between the psychosocial context of a woman's life and her health (RCM 1999, 2001).

The influence of mental health on outcomes was brought sharply into focus by the fact that the leading cause of maternal death in the latest CEMACH report was as a result of psychiatric illness, most deaths being through maternal suicide (Lewis and Drife 2004) (see Chapter 13). As already mentioned inequalities and ethnicity were also risk factors for a greater incidence of maternal and infant mortality. What this means for the focus of care is that, although midwives still have to have a concern for a woman and her baby's physical condition, the social and psychological components of care can no longer be an 'add on' to the physical care (RCM 1999). To save lives midwives have to give equal status to the broader influences on women's well-being, most of which fall under the broader remit of public health. So midwives have to engage with issues around poverty, housing, domestic violence and psychological well-being, and this may involve a change in focus for midwifery care especially in the antenatal and postnatal period. Only by engaging with these issues can midwives ensure that the most vulnerable women are reached and the appropriate services put in place for them.

Multidisciplinary working

The NSF specifically mentions services for women with mental health issues, drug or alcohol use, or disabilities, and women at risk of domestic violence. In addition there is the overriding theme of ensuring that services attend to the needs of deprived women. The role of the midwife in this context is identified within the NSF as one of the following:

- Working as part of a specialist team, e.g. with women who have drug or alcohol issues.
- Ensuring that women who are vulnerable or disadvantaged receive the support that they require or request from the statutory or voluntary services (these may include, for example, advice services or relationship counselling).

On an organizational level the NSF advocates joint working arrangements for vulnerable or disadvantaged women. Examples of joint working may include a fast-track referral system to a perinatal mental health team or working closely with Women's Aid to ensure that support networks are in place for women who disclose domestic violence. The NSF proposes that there are managed care networks for antenatal care with delineation between the specialist services provided in the community and acute/hospital outpatient setting. Within these managed care networks:

> Referrals to and between services are managed through agreed and understood multidisciplinary protocols. The woman's lead carer refers directly and acts as gateway and keeps in regular touch with the woman and the services she receives.
>
> DoH (2004b, p. 45)

In many cases it will be the midwife who is the lead carer for the women and will have the responsibility for maintaining contact with them and the services that they use. The necessity of maintaining contact with a range of services demonstrates the need for continuity of carer for women and families who have contact with a number of different agencies. This way of working reflects the way that some Sure-Start midwives have already developed their role. To enable midwives to establish multidisciplinary working Edwards et al. (2005) advocate the setting up of networks that have a common link through the consultant midwife in public health. Examples of those included in the networks are PCTs, community partnerships, public health networks, Sure-Start midwives, specialist midwives and midwifery team leaders. Through the activity of a consultant midwife the midwifery services are more integrated into local public health initiatives. The scheme outlined above may be one way forward with multidisciplinary working and it is consistent with the stance of the RCM, which proposes moving multidisciplinary working beyond liaison and into the arena of service planning and evaluation (RCM 2001).

BARRIERS TO THE EXPANSION OF AN ENHANCED MIDWIFERY PUBLIC HEALTH ROLE

There are a number of barriers that could limit the possibility of an increased public health role for midwives. First, there is the issue of capacity. A shortage of midwives may be a possible barrier to the restructuring of the maternity services as envisaged in the NSF (RCM 2003). There is evidence that some areas are increasing the public health role of midwives, e.g. through the Sure-Start initiative and the employment of specialist midwives for smoking cessation, teenage mothers or alcohol- and drug-using mothers. However, the implementation is ad hoc and often dependent on external funding (Henderson 2002). As well as the issue of capacity there is also a concern about the running down of the community services in many trusts over the last 10 years. There is increasing unease about the way that the introduction of integrated team midwifery services has often been at the expense of community provision (Anderson 2002). Indeed, a shortage of midwifery staff has been used to justify pulling community staff into hospitals to cover shifts and the abandoning of community provision for home births (Walsh 2004). If staffing levels are low, it means that there is little time to devote to non-medical needs, plus there may not be the capacity to develop the outreach and community services to access women as suggested in CEMACH and the NSF (RCM 2003). However, the need to develop a community-based, proactive service can no longer be ignored because the evidence suggests that the service as it stands is failing some women and contributing to maternal deaths. So it is possible that the NSF will be a catalyst for midwives to think again about the balance between acute and community services.

The lack of expansion in the public health role of midwives may be as result of the ambiguity of midwives themselves. Midwives appear to believe that public health is integral to their role but have definite views about what areas of public health are appropriate for midwifery intervention, e.g. postnatal depression was felt to be appropriate, whereas exercise promotion and cervical screening were not (Lavender et al. 2001). Many of the midwives were wary of taking on tasks that would put extra strain on the capability of the midwifery services to give basic midwifery care or tasks for which they felt inadequately trained. In the present climate these concerns appear legitimate and it is important that an extended midwifery public health role is not used to expand the number of 'tasks' that midwives undertake. There are many public health initiatives that midwifery services can put in place around providing proactive midwifery services for disadvantaged women, and these will benefit public health while retaining the essential core tasks of midwifery (Furber 2000).

Another factor that may limit the feasibility of the public health initiatives suggested in the NSF is the ability of midwives to increase the amount of partnership working. To ensure the best outcome for women with complex needs, the ability for midwives to liaise and work with a wide range of statutory and voluntary services is essential. For this to happen midwives need to overcome the boundaries between different professions and organizations, and some of the Sure-Start initiatives have shown that this is possible given time and patience. In addition, multi-agency and multi-professional approaches need to be developed that are working to achieve common goals (Edwards et al. 2005). It may be easier for midwives to work across boundaries when the profession as a whole is more confident in the parameters of a midwifery public health role and midwifery staff are trained and supported in that role.

A lack of good quality research on effective interventions to improve public health is also a problem when trying to decide how the midwifery public health role should develop (Wanless 2004). One piece of research that is pertinent to the development of a midwifery public health role is that undertaken by Hunt (2004). Hunt's research gives an indication of why disadvantaged women do not access maternity services and her disturbing finding was that it was the attitude of some midwives, and especially hospital midwives, that made women reluctant to access services. These women felt that they were not respected and, although this research does not give hard evidence of interventions that give better outcomes, it gives an indication of how the service could be improved – an improvement that is about a change in the attitude of some midwives towards those in our society who are marginalized.

POSITIVE FACTORS IN THE EXPANSION OF THE PUBLIC HEALTH ROLE OF THE MIDWIFE

There are a number of characteristics in midwifery that will ensure the centrality of a public health role for the profession. It could be argued that public health has always been central to the role of the midwife, either officially or unofficially (Henderson 2002). There have always been many midwives who would ring up the housing office on a family's behalf or help a homeless teenage mother get support from the local social services, alongside most midwives who would support breastfeeding or give advice on good nutrition. So there is potential for the changes envisaged in the NSF to unify both the official and unofficial public health role of the midwife and to build on the existing consensus.

Many midwives feel that they have a special relationship with the women and families for whom they care (Lavender et al. 2001). The special relationship between midwives and their clients is based around a holistic approach to the event of childbirth that acknowledges both the social context of the event and the agency of those involved. So, childbirth is viewed as much more than a clinical event and those involved are ideally viewed as active participants in their care. This view demonstrates that midwifery shares the ethos of public health (Edwards 2005) and that there is a potential for midwifery to define and develop its public health role.

The place that midwives have in their local community, despite its erosion over recent years, means that midwives are ideally situated to help develop community support networks alongside women and their families. *Choosing Health* (DoH 2004a) identifies midwives as having an important role in public health through building social support. Sure-Start initiatives have provided a model in recent years of the potential to increase social capital in an area through promoting client-led groups and peer support. Many of these groups have been devised by midwives alongside other Sure-Start workers in consultation with local women. A shift towards community-led care with midwives visible and contactable in local children's centres, as envisaged by the NSF, will hopefully ensure that midwives are increasingly embedded, and working with the local community to improve public health.

SUMMARY OF KEY POINTS

- There has been an increased acceptance of inequality and deprivation as mediators of health outcomes and as a focus for public health initiatives, as well as an increasing realization that to give more emphasis to the psychosocial context of pregnancy and childbirth can save both lives and money (RCM 2003).
- The latest Government reports, *Choosing Health* (DoH 2004a) and the NSF (DoH 2004b), have an explicit public health agenda that is partially focused on addressing these inequalities in health outcomes.
- For midwives the concentration on deprivation and inequalities has the potential to shift the focus of maternity services back to the community and redress the balance with the acute hospital-based services.
- Although there are barriers to change, not least the shortage of midwives in the UK at the present time, a consensus also exists between some of the fundamentals of midwifery and current Government public health goals. This consensus places midwifery at the centre of the current public health developments.

REFERENCES

Acheson ED (1998) *Independent Inquiry into Inequalities in Health.* London: HMSO.

Anderson T (2002) Integration or disintegration: the scandal of the integration of midwifery services. *MIDIRS Midwifery Digest* **12**: 445–7.

Department of Health (1992) *Health of the Nation: A strategy for health in England.* London: HMSO.

Department of Health (1999) *Saving Lives: Our healthier nation.* London: The Stationery Office.

Department of Health (2001) *Making a Difference: Midwifery action plan*. London: DoH.

Department of Health (2002) *Tackling Health Inequalities: Summary of a cross cutting review*. London: DoH.

Department of Health (2004a) *Choosing Health: Making healthy choices easier*. London: DoH.

Department of Health (2004b) *National Service Framework for Children, Young People and Maternity Services*. London: DoH.

Edwards G, Gordon U, Atherton J (2005) Network approach boosts midwives public health role. *British Journal of Midwifery* **13**: 48–53.

Furber C (2000) An exploration of midwives' attitudes to health promotion. *Midwifery* **16**: 314–22.

Greenwood L (2004) *New Labour NHD Magazine*; available online www.nhs.uk/nhsmagazine/archive/sep04/feat14.asp (accessed June 2005).

Henderson C (2002) The public health role of the midwife. *British Journal of Midwifery* **10**: 268–70.

Hunt S (2004) Poverty, pregnancy and childbirth. *The Practising Midwife* **7**: 12–16.

Lavender T, Bennett N, Blundell J, Malpass L (2001) Midwives' views on redefining midwifery 1: Health promotion. *British Journal of Midwifery* **9**: 666–70.

Leap N, Hunter B (1993) *The Midwife's Tale: An oral history from handywoman to professional midwife*. London: Scarlet Press.

Lewis G, Drife J (2004) *Confidential Enquiry into Maternal and Child Health: Why mothers Die 2000–2002*. London: RCOG.

Palmer G, Carr J, Kenway P (2004) *Monitoring Poverty and Social Exclusion*. London: New Policy Institute/Joseph Rowntree Foundation.

Royal College of Midwives (1999) *Position Paper No. 24: The Midwife's Role in Public Health*. London: RCM.

Royal College of Midwives (2001) *Midwives and the New NHS. Paper 4: Public Health*. London: RCM.

Royal College of Midwives (2003) *Response to Securing Good Health for the Whole Population*. London: RCM.

Walsh D (2004) Home birth, staffing and acute services. *British Journal of Midwifery* **12**: 616.

Wanless D (2004) *Securing Good Health for the Whole Population: Final report*. London: HMSO.

2 HEALTH PROMOTION AND THE MIDWIFE

JAN BOWDEN

Midwives are, by their very nature, promoters of health. Health promotion is not an extended role of the midwife but a core competency. As the lead professional for most of the care provided by the maternity services in the UK, the midwife is in an ideal position to extend support to pregnant and delivered women and their families, and to provide a service that helps parents to access information and use it effectively to nurture the health of their family. They also have an important role in bringing to public attention those health issues that are beyond the scope of individuals to change, such as social and environmental factors. These factors have major implications in undermining health and require community action in order to improve public health for everyone. This chapter, using relevant evidence, looks at the concepts and influences on health and the needs and goals of health promotion. In addition the holistic approach of salutogenesis is discussed and applied to a midwifery context.

CONCEPTS OF HEALTH

Health can mean different things to different people. There are generally thought to be three main concepts:

1. The first is considered the medical concept where people identify that health is not 'being unwell or ill'. This is where there is an absence of illness and disease. It can be argued that this is the predominant view in our health-care service, which is principally designed towards avoiding or overcoming pathogens or stopping disease progression. This is considered by many to be a limited concept which may cause difficulties when promoting health (Ewles and Simnett 2003).

2. The second is described as the 'functional' view of health where individuals identify health as 'being able to do the things you need to do'. This is often the concept of health used by people who already have an issue affecting their health and is used when discussing health in relation to elderly people or those with a disability (Cowley 2002). This view leads to

questioning of society's ability to adjust and act in response to those whose 'function' is impaired by age or disability, despite technology that gets around many of these 'functional' dilemmas (French 1993).

3. The final concept is 'feeling good about yourself'. This suggests how individuals feel about themselves, irrespective of debilitation or disease progression, or the environment in which they find themselves.

The World Health Organization (WHO) used all three concepts as the underlying basis of their constitution in 1946, when it stated that health is 'a state of complete physical, mental and social well-being, and not merely the absence of disease or infirmity' (WHO 1946, p. 2). This has been judged as being somewhat 'rose tinted' in its nature but, to its merit, it does integrate these main concepts of health and identifies that health can be viewed differently by individuals and groups; this needs a great deal of consideration when instigating projects and activities that promote or maintain the health of the population.

The twentieth century has seen the rise in (and some say the return to) the concept of holism in health. This theory is underpinned by the belief that health is multidimensional. The physical, sexual, emotional, mental, social and spiritual aspects of health are interlinked and co-dependent. Therefore an insult or hurt to one aspect of a person's health will have ramifications for all the other aspects (Hancock 2000). Health is also affected by a multitude of external factors such as wealth, education, housing, employment and social networks. This holistic view of health has led to a new approach in health promotion called salutogenesis, which the Royal College of Midwives (RCM) is using in its campaign for normal birth (RCM 2002).

Reflection – 1

- Reflect upon your own concept(s) of health.
- Do they fit into any of the concepts above?

The concept of health can be a particularly complex one for midwives. To be in a state of 'complete … well-being' is hard enough to achieve for most people, but pregnancy and birth are a particular time in a woman's life noted for physical, sexual, emotional, mental, spiritual and social change, and where the limits of 'normality' are exceptionally difficult to set. A further issue is that for many midwives the environment in which they work identifies pregnancy and birth as a 'non-healthy' condition (except perhaps in retrospect, when the 'danger' of birth has been overcome). If a midwife's primary role is detecting and helping to correct ill-health or abnormality, this means that deviations from this predefined and narrow outline of normality will need to be continually looked for and, with extreme vigilance, some will almost certainly be found (Crafter 1997).

However, if childbirth is seen as a normal physiological event, the midwife is likely to have a much broader concept of health and health promotion. In this second situation, the midwife's role will be quite different from that mentioned above. It means moving away from a basically active diagnostic role to a supportive, more 'hands-off' role, facilitating rather than administering. Most midwives probably work somewhere in the middle of this continuum – intervening to help nature along rather than dominating it – and requesting assistance when things are not running smoothly or a medical opinion is required.

THE INFLUENCES ON HEALTH

When looking at health one must look at the influences of health. The factors that can affect health and health promotion can do so in a positive or a negative way and are explored in more depth in Chapter 3. It is rare for health to be purely down to good fortune. A state of good or poor health has been shown to be the result of a combination of factors that are biological, social and/or environmental in their nature (Figure 2.1).

Age, sex and hereditary influences can determine an individual's predisposition to an illness or disease, and they are by and large unalterable. Although with strides in genetics, an individual can, in certain circumstances, be made aware of potential illness and disease and be offered help in preventing it or limiting its effects, e.g. for a condition that is not treatable such as sickle-cell disease, pregnant women and their partners are now offered a screening test and a pathway of care if the results show that both parents carry the trait. Possibly the biggest influences on health are social

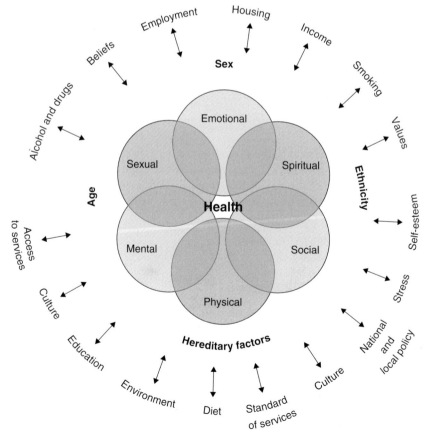

FIGURE 2.1 *Dimensions of health and influencing factors*

and environmental. Research over the last 35 years has provided us with a large quantity of data to show that those who have a high level of income, a better working environment, superior housing, and a greater social network and support have a better level of health, better access to services and a better standard of services when they are ill than those who do not (Tudor-Hart 1971, Townsend and Davidson 1988, Dahlgren and Whitehead 1991, Acheson 1998, Graham 2000, Davey et al. 2001).

More recent data have shown that behavioural and cultural influences also affect health. Lifestyle behaviour and one's ability to assess health risk and make a healthier option make a compelling argument when discussing the influences on health (Dufty 2005). It indicates that, as individuals, we each have responsibility for our own health. An inactive health promoter, lazy primary care trust (PCT) or disinterested government could of course use this as an option for potential blame, by legitimizing their reasons why their health-promoting skills or strategies are ineffective through blame of the individual. It must be made clear that the healthier option is only the healthier option when the 'playing field' of health is flat. Social and environmental influences will shape an individual's ability to undertake assessment of health risks and sway the ability to make the healthier choice. Unfortunately those with the greatest number of inequalities will predominantly be those individuals who make poor health risk assessment and the unhealthier choice (see Chapter 3).

WHAT IS HEALTH PROMOTION?

Activity – 1

Consider what you understand by the term 'health promotion' by writing your own definition.

The concept of health promotion has emerged with the increasing realization in our society that health can and should be improved for everyone, and that our health is one of our most valuable personal assets, as well as an asset for society. Your definition in the above activity may have included some of the following concepts of health promotion:

- Facets from the dimensions of health, i.e. physical, sexual, emotional, mental, spiritual and social health
- Stopping disease progression
- Encouragement of fitness
- Individual, community and/or societal activities
- Health-related education
- Attainment of an individual/community health potential.

It would not be surprising if your definition focused largely on healthy lifestyle issues, because this is a very common elucidation of the term 'health promotion'. It is often used interchangeably with health education but health promotion is so much more than just educating people and communities about health. It would be a huge misconception to limit the term to just 'spreading the word' about healthier lifestyles.

The WHO in 1984 produced the following definition of health promotion:

> Health promotion is the process of enabling people to increase control over, and to improve their health …. Health promotion is a positive concept emphasizing social and personal resources, as well as physical capacities. Therefore, health promotion is not just the responsibility of the health sector, but goes beyond healthy lifestyles to well being …
>
> WHO (1984, p. 5)

The WHO went on to encompass this definition into a major health promotion initiative called *Health for All in the 21st Century* (WHO 1999). This initiative had as its main objective the reduction of health inequalities *within* nations and a reduction of the health inequality gap *between* nations. It clearly recognizes that health promotion involves rallying societal, governmental and, indeed, global responsibility for the health of individuals and communities.

For this to occur the term 'health promotion' must be considered as an umbrella term that encompasses other activities that facilitate the promotion of health (Figure 2.2).

Health promotion must also acknowledge the role of the individual, community and society in nurturing awareness, social support and the development of autonomy and empowerment of all its members, as well as making health reachable for all. These are seen as crucial if health is to be improved in all of society's members, including (and most importantly) those who are deemed socially excluded and least able to access information and services and/or to seek actively 'the healthier option'; this may include young teenage mothers, those women and families living in poverty, homeless individuals and ethnic minority groups.

Health promotion is an activity requiring the participation of all 'stakeholders' – those who have a vested interest in the promotion of health – in order to be successful. As stated by the WHO (1984, 1999) it is important to highlight that it is not just the health sector that is a stakeholder but also the Government, social services, education, employment, housing, utilities, police, legal services and environment; of equal importance are the service users, the people whose health is being promoted. User inclusion is vital for the success of a health promotion activity

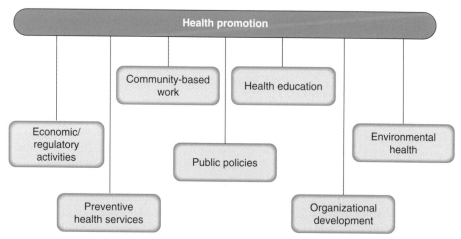

FIGURE 2.2 *Activities encompassed within health promotion. (Adapted from Ewles and Simnett 2003.)*

or project, e.g. when initiating a project to improve the health of pregnant women on an inner city estate, the women's opinions and knowledge are vital, to ensure that the project being developed is sensitive to the reality in which these women and their families live. To design and implement a project developed by policy-makers and health professionals alone without such user involvement is destined to failure. This is because the women will have things done to them by outsiders, rather than having their real needs respected, valued and addressed.

Failure to involve users will lead to any benefits that are seen unlikely to be sustained over a long period of time (Department of Health (DoH) 1999a). For health promotion to be successful it must be sustainable and have longevity. Health promotion therefore must understand and respond to people's needs. The same is true of the health promotion activities undertaken by a midwife working one to one with her clients; exploration of each woman's knowledge and opinions, and respect for them, are crucial if the woman is to feel that these health-promoting activities and indeed her midwifery care are of value to her (Milburn 1996).

Health promotion can be effective only if it is understood that health depends on a multitude of factors with complicated and, as yet, poorly understood interrelationships. The most apparent of these factors includes people's values, attitudes and behaviour, and the relationship between them and their health (see Chapter 6). It is not essential, as well as probably not being possible, for the health promoter to understand every aspect of individual's relationship between their values, attitude and behaviour, and their health, but it is necessary to be aware that a relationship exists and that health is affected by circumstances that are neither straightforward nor quick to change.

SALUTOGENESIS: A HOLISTIC APPROACH TO HEALTH PROMOTION IN MIDWIFERY?

There has been a move away from the preventive/medical model of health and health promotion because it is clear that individuals do not simply stop doing things because they are informed of how bad it is for them. If that were the case breastfeeding rates would rocket and smoking in pregnancy would be a thing of the past. The concept of holism in health has taken on more importance in recent years and with it a more holistic approach to health promotion has been pursued. This holistic approach to health promotion would fundamentally assess health factors and coping strategies rather than assess for illness and risk factors.

Salutogenesis may offer this approach, developed by Aaron Antonovsky, a medical sociologist; Antonovsky identified that health is a state of flux which is negotiated throughout an individual's life. Sometimes an individual can negotiate it well and at other times not so well. It is dependent on the individual's ability to cope and the resources and support available (Antonovsky 1993). Although not instantly identifiable as user friendly, the constituent parts of salutogenesis are, for all intents and purposes, very applicable to midwifery and the midwife's role in health promotion.

This approach is at the opposite end of the spectrum to the medical approach and its pathogenic route. It considers the creation of well-being by looking at successful coping strategies and health. It encourages the examination of the wider picture in order to identify the health problem and the disorder that it causes, and seeks out the coping strategies and resources required to improve health or prevent further deterioration (RCM 2002). The resources may be internal, e.g. the cognitive ability to cope with a newborn infant, or external such as housing or employment, and are important for the growth and continuance of a 'sense of coherence', which Antonovsky feels is synonymous with health. The more enhanced the 'sense of coherence' the better the individual's ability to employ cognitive, affective and behaviour strategies, which will improve coping mechanisms and maintain well-being. Antonovsky (1993) identifies three basic necessities for successfully coping:

1. Meaningfulness: life's trials and tribulations are worthy of commitment and life has some emotional sense to it. The individual must see coping as a desirable skill.
2. Manageability: the individual believes that support and resources are effortlessly found and straightforwardly accessible when needed.
3. Comprehensibility: the level to which an individual organizes his or her world to bring understanding, meaning, order and consistency to it.

The extent to which these necessities develop is dependent on the individual's sense of self and socialization. Salutogenesis considers social capital and health capital as determining factors in developing a 'sense of coherence'. Teenage mothers and refugee women can be seen as two examples of clients who may have these basic necessities either undeveloped or weakened, and this approach offers a midwife some understanding as to how these clients' ability to cope and make healthier life choices could be impacted upon.

The approach goes some way to scrutinize why certain groups within our society are disadvantaged in their health options, their ability to access the care and the standard of the services that they receive, and identifies a route by which resources and support are developed and used. All of this enhances the midwife's knowledge and skills when promoting health on a one-to-one basis with a client and when working and developing her public health role and ability to function in partnership working (Cowley and Billing 1999). (Partnership working is discussed in Chapter 9.)

NEEDS IN HEALTH PROMOTION

The meaning of 'need' is an interesting one where health promotion is concerned. A need is a prerequisite when initiating health promotion. Therefore if there is no need there can be no health promotion. For a lengthy period within health promotion, the prerequisite need has predominantly been set by the health-care professionals, usually the doctors and the Government. This kind of need is a desirable or expected standard, which is usually laid down in the form of a policy or recommendation that more often than not comes with a target to be reached within a set period of time, e.g. the *National Strategy for Sexual Health and HIV* (DoH 2001). However, evidence suggests that needs identified by users are often more successfully met, especially when all stakeholders have played a full and equal part (DoH 1999a, Kemshall and Littlechild 2000). So how are needs in health promotion defined?

The *Oxford Concise Dictionary of Current English* (Allen 1993) states that a need is 'a want or requirement'. Bradshaw (1972) attempted the difficult task of breaking down the concept of social need into more measurable units, in order to assess requirements more rationally than can be done without such a quantifiable framework. In his now classic and frequently quoted taxonomy he identified four types of need:

1. Normative need: a desirable/expected standard laid down by the professional, often in the form of a policy or recommendation.

2. Felt need or what people actually want: this is the most nebulous of Bradshaw's needs and may eventually become an expressed need.
3. Expressed need, i.e. the service requested/demanded by an individual, group or community.
4. Comparative need: occurs where the recipients of a service are compared to assess gaps and inequality in service provision. The need is to bring about equality and fairness.

These concepts are clearly useful in assessing health needs, by making them more definable and less abstract. However, this taxonomy also allows the midwife to examine the difficulties that arise with these definitions. A normative need can be seen as a 'top-down' approach, which is not always the ideal in health promotion. A further issue is that this is a value judgement made by a professional and, as we know, professionals may contradict each other over what is a desirable/expected standard. In addition, a normative need identified by a professional may vary considerably from the need of the client. A felt need may be inflated or limited, depending on the knowledge of the individual or group that is communicating this felt need, and may or may not develop into an expressed need, which may be a result of a lack of opportunity, motivational issues or poor assertiveness skills on the part of the individual or group. The expressed need can have its own difficulties, in that it may be in opposition to an already identified normative need and therefore conflict may arise between the expressed and normative needs (Ewles and Simnett 2003). With a comparative need there is a comparison between two different groups, some receiving a health promotion activity or project and some not – the latter identified as in need. There is the possibility that this may lead to 'positive' discrimination for those in the need group until that group reaches the same level of those already in receipt of the health promotion activity or project.

Activity – 2

The concept of social need

1. Normative need: How are the normative needs of women formalized in your work setting? (If there is a 'standard setting' or 'clinical quality assurance' team in your place of work they will have details.) What normative needs has your area of practice formally accepted?
2. Felt need: Have there been any felt needs expressed by your clients either individually or as a group? How did you react to this and was it possible for it to become an expressed need?
3. Expressed need: Which organizations do you identify as being the most vocal in demanding changes in health provision for maternity care and young families? Have they made any difference in the service provision that you see around you? If yes, what are these differences?
4. Comparative need: Do the women you observe accessing maternity care receive comparative care? What general and individual factors affect comparable care, or prevent its deliverance? Access information about another maternity unit. Do women in your maternity unit have comparable access to, for example, fetal screening tests?

However, just as health is not a state that can be measured with precision, nor are health needs straightforward. In assessing such needs, the midwife will also need to consider other issues beyond those identified by Bradshaw. Scope of practice and the boundaries of the midwife's position, together with the degree of autonomy, will all play a part, along with some degree of dependency on the midwife's line manager, e.g. the setting up of a breastfeeding workshop or a teenage mothers' parenting group may be considered by the line manager as a health promotion activity for a midwife, but becoming involved in educational work around sexual health within local schools may, sadly, not be. Another consideration must look at whether the need being assessed is reactive – responding to an expressed need – or proactive – where the midwife initiates the need. Pressures from strong vocal groups of women may introduce bias in how needs are agreed and generate pressure to react, perhaps to the detriment of other women. Acting proactively may mean saying no to an expressed need and initiating a professional's normative need (Ewles and Simnett 2003). The issue of whose needs come first – the user or the provider – must also be borne in mind when a midwife sets out to develop a health promotion project because this may give rise to conflict between the two, e.g. a user might request a Saturday breastfeeding workshop because child care, parking and attendance are easier to achieve than on a weekday, but the provider may not be able to facilitate this need because of difficulties with staffing, which is usually at lower levels at a weekend. Further consideration about who decides that there is a need and what the grounds are for taking this decision must also be identified as part of the health needs assessment process (Ewles and Simnett 2003).

THE AIMS OF HEALTH PROMOTION

Once a health needs assessment has been completed and a need identified, the next stage of planning is the identification of what is going to be achieved by a health promotion project. A whole plethora of words has been used to describe what is to be achieved – aims, goals, mission statement, purpose, targets, objectives and outcomes, to name but a few. But whatever they are called, it is vital to stress their importance because they indicate what the project expects to achieve. They are important because they allow evaluation to take place, an evaluation that will measure either success or failure. It is therefore crucial that the aims are simple, attainable and crystal clear, as this will allow the evaluation of what has occurred against what the health promoter wanted to occur, and from this the project will hopefully be judged a success.

Aims usually revolve around the themes of process and product. The 'process' of health promotion involves the way in which people gain information and understanding, and how their decision-making skills are enhanced in using or disregarding the information as they see fit. The 'process' of health promotion, even when aims are specific, is notoriously tricky to measure. The 'product' of health promotion, or the end result, is often not quantifiable and is therefore difficult to measure, without involving significantly large numbers of people, and the multitude of other factors that could lead to such a result may not be taken into account (Crafter 1997) (see Chapter 5).

Teenage pregnancy is a good example to use when formulating the aims of a health promotion activity. In terms of process, a midwife may decide that the goals are to raise awareness of sexual issues among first-time teenage mothers, and provide a forum where relationships, personal values and contraceptive methods can be openly discussed and explored. The product aim after such an activity may be to increase the length of time between the first and second baby.

The aims of a health promotion activity or project should reflect the needs of the users, not those of the midwife. In raising awareness of sexual issues with teenagers, some of them may choose to plan their pregnancies in seemingly dire social circumstances, although it could be argued that this is about poor educational opportunity and socioeconomic factors, rather than true choice (Teenage Pregnancy Unit (TPU) 2003). It may be difficult for the midwife to accept individuals' decisions about their lives, but this does not allow the midwife to decide what is best for these young women. The teenage mothers themselves should also define the issues because they know best the pressures, problems and realities in their lives, and they hold the key to how these areas can be addressed best (Social Exclusion Unit (SEU) 1999, Health Development Agency 2004).

The midwife would have the knowledge to realize that just one-to-one or one-to-small group activities will have relatively little impact on the deep-seated reasons of why first-time teenage mothers fall pregnant quickly with a second child. Many of the issues in this example are best dealt with at a community level rather than with individuals, addressing the issues of education and socioeconomic problems that affect first-time teenage mothers (SEU 1999, TPU 2003). Therefore, the midwife's health promotion activity will incorporate working with other agencies (partners), e.g. Sure Start. The Sure-Start and Sure-Start Plus programmes, in which many midwives across the UK are now involved, are excellent illustrations of how the above example can work in practice through work with individuals and in partnership with other agencies. Sure Start has given users an equal stake within the project, has midwives as one of the lead practitioners involved and demonstrates the midwives' capabilities for working in partnership (DoH 1999b, Wiggins et al. 2003).

SUMMARY OF KEY POINTS

- Health means different things to different people. It incorporates a delicate combination of factors, some individual and some societal. Adequate definitions of health should incorporate cultural and environmental overtones. If pregnancy and childbirth are not seen as a normal, cultural and/or family-centred event, this has negative implications for the role and responsibilities of the midwife as a health promoter.
- Health is one of our most valuable personal assets. It can be improved for many women, particularly the increasing numbers who are deemed to be socially excluded.
- Health and health promotion are moving away from the preventive/medical model to a more holistic one, in which assessment of health factors and coping strategies rather than assessment of illness and risk factors is preferred.
- Salutogenesis can provide the necessary holistic approach to health promotion that midwives need to provide them with the knowledge and skills to work in their usual health promoting roles, as well as developing their role in public health and partnership working.
- Health promotion is so much more than just educating people and communities about health. It would be a huge misconception to limit the term to just 'spreading

the word' about healthier lifestyles. Health promotion involves rallying societal, governmental and, indeed, global responsibility for the health of individuals and communities. For this to occur, the term 'health promotion' must be considered as an umbrella term, which integrates other activities that facilitate the promotion of health.

■ Health promotion must acknowledge the complicated interrelationships between socioeconomic and environmental factors, and health. Individual behaviour is not the only cause of ill-health, and therefore the general health of society will not be greatly improved by health promotion specifically targeted at individuals.

■ The focus for improving public health must be on a social policy that is sensitive to the needs and circumstances of all groups in society, not just the most vocal. To be effective, midwives must work with women as equal stakeholders.

REFERENCES

Acheson D (1998) *Independent Inquiry in to Inequalities in Health*. London: The Stationery Office.

Allen RE (ed.) (1993) *Oxford Concise Dictionary of Current English*, 8th edn. Oxford: Oxford University Press.

Antonovsky A (1993) The structure and properties of the sense of coherence scale. *Social Science and Medicine* **36**: 725–33.

Bradshaw J (1972) The concept of social need. *New Society* **19**: 640–3.

Cowley S (ed.) (2002) *Public Health in Policy and Practice: A sourcebook for health visitors and community nurses*. London: Baillière Tindall.

Cowley S, Billing J (1999) Resources revisited: Salutogenesis from a lay perspective. *Journal of Advanced Nursing* **29**: 994–1004.

Crafter H (ed.) (1997) Health promotion and the midwife. In: *Health Promotion in Midwifery Principles and Practice*. London: Arnold.

Dahlgren G, Whitehead M (1991) *Policies and Strategies to Promote Social Equity in Health*. Stockholm: Institute for Future Studies.

Davey B, Gray A, Seale C (2001) *Health And Disease – A reader*, 3rd edn. Buckingham: Open University Press.

Department of Health (1999a) *Patient and Public Involvement in the New NHS*. London: DoH.

Department of Health (1999b) *Sure Start*. London: DoH.

Department of Health (2001) *The National Strategy for Sexual Health and HIV*. London: DoH.

Dufty J (2005) 'They have only themselves to blame ...' Understanding the political, psychosocial and environmental drivers that power the trend for unhealthy lifestyle behaviours in deprived communities. *MIDIRS Midwifery Digest* **15**: 115–20.

Ewles L, Simnett I (2003) *Promoting Health: A practical guide*, 5th edn. London: Baillière Tindall.

French S (1993) Disability, impairment or something in between? In: Swain J, Finkelstein V, French S, Oliver M (eds), *Disabling Barriers – Enabling Environments*. London: Sage.

Graham H (2000) *Understanding Health Inequalities*. Buckingham: Open University Press.

Hancock B (2000) Are nursing theories holistic? *Nursing Standard* **14**: 37–41.

Health Development Agency (2004) *Teenage Pregnancy: An overview of the research evidence*. London: HDA.

Kemshall H, Littlechild R (2000) *User Involvement and Participation in Social Care*. London: Jessica Kingsley.

Milburn M (1996) The importance of lay theorizing for health promotion research and practice. *Health Promotion International* **11**: 41–6.

Royal College of Midwives (2002) *What is Salutogenesis?* London: RCM.

Social Exclusion Unit (1999) *Teenage Pregnancy: A Report by the Social Exclusion Unit.* London: The Stationery Office.

Teenage Pregnancy Unit (2003) *Sure Start Plus Pilot Programme – National Evaluation of Sure Start Plus.* London: Teenage Pregnancy Unit.

Townsend P, Davidson N (1988) The Black Report. In: Townsend P, Davidson N, Whitehead M (eds) *In equalities in Health: The Black Report and the health divide.* Harmondsworth: Penguin, pp. 29–213.

Tudor-Hart J (1971) The inverse care law. *Lancet* **i**: 405.

Wiggins M, Austerberry H, Rosato M, Sawtell M, Oliver S (2003) *Sure Start Plus National Evaluation Service Delivery Study: Interim Findings.* London: University of London.

World Health Organization (1946) *Constitution.* New York: WHO.

World Health Organization (1984) *Health Promotion: A WHO discussion document on the Concepts and Principles.* (Reprinted in: *Journal of the Institute of Health Education* (1985) **23** (1): 11–14.)

World Health Organization (1999) *Health 21 – Health for All in the 21st Century.* Copenhagen: WHO Regional Office for Europe.

FURTHER READING

Acheson D (1998) *Independent Inquiry in to Inequalities in Health.* London: The Stationery Office.

Department of Health (2004) *National Service Framework for Children, Young People, and Maternity Services.* London: DoH.

Wanless D (2004) *Securing Good Health for the Whole Population: Final report.* Norwich: The Stationery Office.

3 FACTORS AFFECTING HEALTH PROMOTION

HEATHER FINLAY

Making people aware of their ability to make healthy choices is problematic. There are a number of different approaches to trying to help people change their behaviour and make healthier choices. It is worth identifying the two main approaches to promoting healthy behaviours before looking specifically at the impact of gender on the ability to make healthy choices. The first approach is the health education model. Traditionally this model has concentrated on changing individual behaviour. The second main approach to changing behaviour is the health promotion model, which differs from health education models by looking beyond the individual and placing health in a sociopolitical framework (Whitehead and Russell 2004). There is increasing recognition that a person's health and health choices are affected by factors such as education, income, employment, environment, access to health services and social support (Wurst et al. 2002).

An acknowledgement that health promotion needs to look beyond the individual is particularly important for women. The lives of women influence the way that they are able to make healthy choices, and strategies to encourage women to change their behaviour that do not take this into account have poor outcomes. So, what is it about being a woman that makes it difficult to utilize health education and make healthier choices? This chapter considers the mediating factors that may influence the response of women to health education.

WHAT MAKES WOMEN DIFFERENT?

The health education model makes a number of 'commonsense' assumptions about the way that women may be influenced by health education. If women are given the knowledge in an accessible way, it is assumed that they will make a rational choice and change their behaviour, and they will act in ways that serve their own interests and their actions will reproduce their understanding of the causes and nature of ill-health (Currie and Weisenburg 2003). The process of making a decision about whether or not to make a positive health choice is therefore seen as a simple cost–benefit analysis, where the woman can rationally weigh up the 'cost' or difficulty of changing her behaviour against the 'benefit' of changing her behaviour (however long term or vague that benefit may be).

However, regardless of gender, there is evidence that it is too simplistic to assume that the health education information offered is accepted unconditionally. We know that health education information is interpreted and this interpretation depends on existing beliefs (Joffe 2002). So, for both men and women it would be unwise to assume that making healthy choices results from rational and objective decision-making (Whitehead and Russell 2004). It would seem that there is more going on. If health education does not necessarily change behaviour by changing beliefs, there is a need to look beyond this simplistic relationship and consider the health promotion model. The key to exploring this model is to include mediating factors and their part in explaining health behaviours. There are mediating factors that are specific to women and will influence their response to health education or health promotion. These situational factors are less a product of women's life choices and more a product of their life chances or circumstances. These life chances or circumstances will be a reflection of women's interaction between themselves and among their family, community and environment (Currie and Weisenburg 2003). In most cases these life circumstances override lifestyle choices and are a major influence on women's ability to make healthy choices.

FAMILY, HOME AND EXPECTATIONS

One mediating factor that may make a woman less or more able to make healthy choices is when caring for a family, either with or without a partner. Gender stereotypes usually designate women as the carer within a household. This reflects a cultural acceptance that it is more natural for women to be 'nurturing'. Women's normal responsibilities within the home can be extensive and include preparing nutritious meals, caring for family members (including elderly and disabled individuals) and keeping the home clean. As well as this women may be expected to travel long distances to take children to school, to treat common illnesses and to maintain the emotional well-being of the household members (Currie and Weisenburg 2003). For women who have paid employment outside the home, this can lead to role conflict and stress as a woman tries to be a 'superwoman/supermum'.

Ball et al. (2003) looked at the feasibility of healthy eating and physical activity for young women and illustrated how family and home commitments can limit a woman's ability to make healthy choices. The study questioned 463 women aged between 18 and 32 years about the perceived feasibility of adopting a healthy diet and exercise regime and they found that:

> In particular, changes in a young women's domestic situation as they leave the family home, enter a *de facto* partnership or marriage, or have children are likely to have a major influence on their ability to adopt or adhere to healthy behaviours.
>
> Ball et al. (2003, p. 434)

Women with children found leisure-time physical activity and using walking or cycling as a mode of transport less feasible than other groups of women, but they found fruit and vegetable consumption to be more feasible than other groups.

So, while the women with children in the Ball et al. study may not make time to exercise for its own sake, they will take on board messages about keeping their children and partner healthy through increased fruit and vegetable intake. It is common for women to put their own needs second to those of the family, especially when there is a limited family income (Hunt 2004a). Although a woman may be the principal motivator for those in the family to seek treatment or make healthier choices, there may not be anyone in the family to encourage the woman to do the same. In practical terms a woman may put her own health at risk to maintain the family. One example of this is setting a high threshold of illness to avoid having to disrupt the family when a woman's labour is vital (Currie and Weisenburg 2003). A woman may need to see a doctor but her inability to find anyone to take over her caring role may lead to her delaying the visit until it can no longer be avoided. Similarly any time for preventive self-care can be a scarce luxury, so although a woman's knowledge of preventive health choices may be high, her ability to act on them will be limited.

A woman's ability to access services when she has family commitments may be affected by other constraints. One example is the opening times of antenatal clinics (in both the hospital or the community), usually during the day and with little scope for a woman to choose an appointment time. In addition there are rarely crèche or play facilities for children. If a woman has to pick up children from school or cannot face a long wait with a 2 year old, it is easy to see why she may limit her attendance or avoid attending at all. Such a choice may not be a reflection of a woman's knowledge, but rather of her circumstances. There is limited research in this area but it would seem that sociodemographic factors do curtail antenatal care for many women (Rowe and Garcia 2003).

Activity – 1

Think of a situation where you have found it difficult to make a healthy choice, e.g. doing some exercise. What has made it difficult for you? How much are the limiting factors linked to your role as a carer?

WOMEN'S PLACE IN SOCIETY

Although much of the literature on health education acknowledges the complexity of the cost–benefit analysis of making healthy choices, there is little acknowledgement of the role of power and authority in mediating women's decisions to adopt healthier behaviours. The relationship between the genders has changed over recent years in the UK, but for some women there are still issues around power and control. There are women who are marginalized from decision-making, both within a family setting and at a community level. Also some of these women are subject to various forms of physical or sexual violence. This powerlessness may have consequences for women's ability to make choices. The locus of control theory (Tones 1991) suggests that having an external locus of control, where events in one's life are perceived as being governed by powerful others or 'fate', will reduce a person's ability to see the value of trying to change the situation (or health). It has been found that women experiencing domestic violence have feelings of worthlessness and inadequacy, and lack confidence. Women also report an inability to think clearly, or make choices or decisions (Boothroyd 2002). Thus, women disempowered by their situation may feel that it is hopeless to try to adopt healthy choices, even if they are aware of them. This theory has been criticized for placing too much emphasis on the individual at the expense of an understanding of the place of family, community and environment in mediating women's health choices. In practice the choices that women make are probably a result of a number of factors, both psychological and situational.

Powerlessness within a personal or family relationship can manifest itself in many ways, such as lack of financial control, physical or psychological coercion, expectations of women's behaviour or not being permitted to access knowledge around healthier choices. Similarly the decision to seek preventive screening or health care may not be the woman's alone (Currie and Weisenburg 2003). Lack of control over household finances would make it difficult to buy good quality food or even fill prescriptions (except during pregnancy). Lack of money for fares may prevent a woman from attending appointments or attending sporadically. Women who reported violence often booked late for their antenatal care and many did not attend regularly once booked (Lewis 2002).

For many women coping with issues of power and control, their priorities for promoting health may be very different from those of the orthodox health services. Wurst et al. (2002) undertook a qualitative study to explore the family health promotion processes among single mothers with children who had left abusive male partners. The health-promoting factors that were identified for these women were rooted in preventing further intrusion into their life by their violent partners and recreating a safe, nurturing family unit with affordable housing. The prevention of intrusion formed a foundation on which women could then re-build their lives, including promoting their own health and that of their children. Although this would not necessarily be recognized as a fundamental health promotion priority, for these women it certainly is.

Women's responses to health promotion are mediated by their particular experiences and life situations. There are many psychological and practical issues that prevent women from making healthy choices. Also women may have priorities that they see as promoting health which may be outside the remit of the biomedical model of health.

WOMEN AND POVERTY

Women are more vulnerable to poverty than men, especially if they have children. Women's vulnerability is perpetuated by their place in the labour market. The gender pay gap means that women earn less than men when they are in work. Also, women's work is often part-time, low paid and insecure. The Fawcett Society estimates that, in the UK, 4.7 million women earn less than £5 an hour, which is 43 per cent of all employees (Fawcett Society 2005).

Poor wages alongside the high cost of childcare means that many women, even if they are working, are not financially secure. Women who do not work are at risk of poverty by virtue of either being in a low-wage household or being dependent on state benefits (Rosenblatt and Rake 2003). Lone parent families are particularly susceptible to poverty, as are black and ethnic minority women and disabled individuals (Hunt 2004b). It is inevitable that being in poverty challenges a woman's ability to make healthy choices and poverty is another mediating factor in women's response to health promotion.

Women facing such situations are likely to have family and home commitments that override their own health needs and they may also be subject to factors around power and control. In addition being poor brings its own restraints. A lack of money may make it difficult to follow health education guidelines on diet (especially in pregnancy). Living in a deprived area can mean a shortage of local shops – referred to as living in a 'nutritional desert'. Wynn et al.'s (1994) work looked at the difference in diet between women who were on low income and those who had enough money while pregnant. It was found that the diet of poorer women, and especially women who were pregnant and without a partner, differed significantly in major nutrients from those women for whom money was not an issue. Wynn et al.'s findings back up the assertion that when money is short it is the women in households who sacrifice their own basic needs (including food) to make sure that other members of the household do not go without (Rosenblatt and Rake 2003).

A lack of money may also mean that women are unable to take advantage of facilities outside their immediate area (or even inside their immediate area unless they are free). The cost of transport may be prohibitive and the facilities for claiming fares back retrospectively does not solve the problem when there is no money before the journey is started, or if a woman has no recourse to public funds and her status in the UK is unclear.

Hunt (2004b) has also identified that poorer women may find themselves stigmatized within the health system. The women in Hunt's study felt that the midwives judged them by their address and they commonly felt as if they were being 'treated like dirt' or 'something they [the midwives] trod on' (Hunt 2004a, p. 14). Interviews with the midwives confirmed that many of the hospital midwives judge the women from the poorer areas negatively (although the community midwives tended to behave more positively towards the women). The stigmatization of poorer women within the health care system can result in a perception by women that they are receiving substandard care. One woman in Hunt's study said:

> I have changed my GP three times: they won't come out at night. They think that the likes of us aren't worth it. Whatever the problem is the receptionist says bring 'em down to the surgery. That's okay if you've got a car, but how do you bring one sick kid down, wrapped in a blanket with three others in tow.
>
> Hunt (2004b, p. 192)

The feeling that the health system is against them can mean women stop engaging and this may include the area of health promotion.

For many poorer women the messages around better health choices may be at odds with their perceived priorities; an example of this may be smoking cessation. Hunt (2004b) found that for many women smoking was one of the few ways that the women in her study could do something for themselves and find some relaxation. For these women the health risks were not as immediate as the contentment gained from having a cigarette:

> Fags are good to relax. After a hard day with the kids, I like to curl up with a fag. I only smoke when the kids are outside or after they have gone to bed. I know it's not good for them, but it's good for me, it helps me unwind.
>
> Hunt (2004b, p. 200)

Poverty brings many practical limitations to choices, such as an inability to afford a nutritious diet that may make health education messages unrealistic for many women. The constraints of being poor may also mean that women's priorities are at odds with the prevailing health promotion priorities, thus making promotion messages inconsequential in women's everyday lives.

Activity – 2

Imagine you have two children (ages 3 and 1 year) and you are pregnant. The antenatal clinic is an hour's walk away or a half-hour bus ride. At the clinic there is usually a long wait and as your appointment is at 11.30 you will be there over lunchtime; also there is nowhere for the children to play. Think about how the local antenatal clinic services may be reorganized to make your life easier.

BLACK AND ETHNIC MINORITY WOMEN

Black and ethnic minority women will share many of the issues already identified which may restrict their ability to make healthy choices. However, they have additional constraints that may affect their ability both to engage with the health system and to take on the health education messages. The previous section on poverty noted that there was some stereotyping of poorer women within the health service. Stereotypical and racist comments have also been reported by Muslim women while using maternity services (Ali and Burchett 2004). It is possible that black and ethnic minority women may find it difficult to engage with a health system that is seen as threatening, in a similar way to that identified in some of the research around poorer women.

A lack of interpreter services or advocacy support in some areas has been identified by both the Maternity Alliance (Ali and Burchett 2004) and the Royal College of Midwives (RCM 2004) as a problem for black and ethnic minority women. The health system also lacks understanding of cultural norms, which may be a fundamental obstacle to women engaging. The Maternity Alliance (Ali and Burchett 2004) has also highlighted a lack of provision of easily understandable information for women whose first language is not English. This lack of facilities for health education messages to be understood or explained will limit the amount to which healthy choices can be assimilated into women's lives.

FINDING WAYS TO REACH WOMEN

A health promotion approach that can help to tackle some of the situational and environmental barriers that prevent women making healthy choices may be more useful than merely giving information or advice.

Practical change: making healthy choice easier

At a Government level it is increasingly acknowledged that keeping healthy is not just about individual choices but that good or bad health is contingent on a number of factors, including environment, access to services, social support and others

(Department of Health 2003). As women can be especially prone to external influences on their health (e.g. poverty), a broader approach to health promotion will have a disproportionate effect on women's ability to make healthy choices for themselves and their families. There are a number of innovative schemes that have been introduced (some of which are within the author's own practice area) which are designed to make it easier for women to make healthier choices and some of these schemes are outlined below:

- In east London a new bus service has been introduced that goes directly from an area on the edge of the borough (classified as an area of deprivation and where few people have cars) to the local hospital. Before the introduction of the bus service local people had to catch two buses to the nearest hospital and the journey took up to one and a half hours. The travel time to the hospital has been cut by half with the new bus service, and it is hoped that if will make it easier for people to attend their hospital appointments.
- Local cooperative schemes are providing low-cost fruit and vegetable boxes. In some areas these boxes are available at local schools and health centres. The provision of low-cost fruit and vegetable boxes makes it easier for women to provide their families (and themselves) with a more balanced diet. In areas where there is little choice in the food available to buy and travel to the nearest large shops is expensive, these boxes may be the only access to fresh fruit and vegetables. Some areas are combining the boxes with cookery clubs where women can learn to cook seasonal produce and introduce them to their family.
- A drop-in family planning clinic (including pregnancy testing) set up locally and timed to be convenient for women picking up and dropping off children at school. This clinic will also have a midwife dropping in to ensure that women who are pregnant can access the maternity services easily. The clinic is in an area where a disproportionate number of women access the maternity services late in their pregnancy.
- In the north-west of England the timing of an antenatal clinic was changed to ensure that Muslim women could attend during Ramadan. It had been noted that women found it hard to attend antenatal appointments as a result of fasting and having to prepare meals early in the morning and late at night. The alternative timing of the clinics appeared to increase the number of women attending (Pearce and Mayho 2004).

As can be seen from the list above, there are ways to make it easier for women to make healthier choices and in its broadest sense that is health promotion. It could be argued that it is unreasonable to expect women to make healthy choices, in response to increased knowledge or awareness, without practical changes. However, practical changes and increased knowledge or awareness may still not be sufficient for some women to feel that they can make healthier choices. Also influencing a woman's ability to make healthier choices is how much women feel that they can take control and effect change and the ability to do this depends on how empowered women feel themselves to be.

Empowerment

Empowerment can be defined in a number of different ways and circumstances. Definitions can apply to whole communities or to individuals. The commonalities within definitions of empowerment involve the ability to take control, effect change and improve the quality of life for those involved (Becker et al. 2004). At a community level, empowerment may lead to environmental or service change. An example of this might be a local community coming together to lobby the local primary care trust for a birth centre in their area. On an individual level, empowerment may allow an individual to develop her own way of exercising control over her thoughts, feelings and actions, and begin to acquire a perceived self-efficacy (Becker et al. 2004). This means that a person develops a belief in her own ability to make changes in her life, moving from an external to an internal locus of control. An example of this could be a woman deciding to approach her general practitioner about a long-standing medical problem.

Empowerment is acknowledged as being part of health promotion. Empowerment can work alongside practical changes to promote the achievement of more positive health choices (Peterson and Hughey 2004), e.g. within a community health promotion initiative a community should identify its own health needs. Therefore the initiative that is put in place will reflect the priorities of that community and may achieve more. However, there may be difficulties in implementing community involvement. The process of communities empowering themselves involves service providers allowing decision-making and problem-solving to be a shared responsibility. It may be difficult for health-care providers to appreciate the expertise and abilities of women and their communities. Health-care providers may also struggle with not being the one who automatically provides the solutions (Portela and Santarelli 2003).

The Sure-Start initiative is an example of an attempt to involve a community in local health initiatives and health promotion. In the way the initiative is set up currently, Sure-Start projects involve elements of community empowerment. Although the projects have Government set targets, the way in which these targets are implemented is decided by a board of local parents, voluntary organizations and other interested parties. Indeed one of the Sure-Start principles is that the projects should be community driven but professionally coordinated. The majority of the Sure-Start services have concentrated their efforts on health and education promotion for women and children, although there is an increasing inclusion of partners and other carers in the projects. Many of the services include groups led not by professionals but by the participants themselves. One example is a teenage mothers' club in the north-west of England (Gostling 2003). Midwives noticed that teenagers were not attending the existing groups for pregnant women or mothers and babies. By talking to the young women, the midwives discovered that some of the pregnant teenagers were meeting at each other's houses because they felt that the existing services did not cater for their needs. Many young women in the area were missing out on health promotion while pregnant or as new mothers. In addition young women were under-using the services on offer. In response to this, funding was found to set up the teenage club. Once set up, the club was client led, with an emphasis on peer support and education. The club has also formed links with the local teenage pregnancy working group and has proved the catalyst for an increased profile for the needs of pregnant teenagers within the maternity services. The experience in the north-west illustrates how a community (in this case pregnant teenagers) can begin empowering themselves given the appropriate tools, such as funding, a venue and support from health professionals.

Not only do groups, such as the teenager group discussed above, encourage empowerment; they can also improve social capital in areas where the local populations may have changed profile and social capital may be reduced. Social capital is defined as:

> Both formal and informal reciprocal links among people in all sorts of family, friendship, business and community networks.
>
> Lynch et al. (2000, p. 404)

It is felt by some that increased social capital, characterized by bonding, linking, participation and trust, within a community setting can have benefits for health and can increase the impact of health promotion (Lynch et al. 2000). However, there is also some debate about the characteristics of social capital and the different potentials for the various forms of social capital to improve the uptake of healthier choices (Baum and Ziersch 2003). But, overall, an increase in social networks and social support appears to benefit women.

For some women involvement in groups can increase their feelings of empowerment and possibly contribute to social capital in their community. It appears that empowerment is fostered for women in group situations, which include participation and connectedness, rather than just activities (Peterson and Hughey 2004). Groups that include peer support and/or a sense of a group working together will therefore be more suited to women's empowerment. However, empowerment can also take place at an individual level. As joining groups is not an option for some women, whether through choice, isolation or illness, empowerment for these women can be facilitated individually. The MOMobile programme in the USA utilizes local advocates to work with low-income mothers in the local community (Becker et al. 2004). The aim of the project is for the advocates to provide support, health promotion and referrals where needed. The advocates identified themselves as helping to empower women through the encouragement of self-determination, decision-making and self-sufficiency:

> A client comes with no ideas what her rights are, about everything, and then you educate them or teach them and that's when we are making a difference. And then afterwards when we form a relationship and watch them on their own strengthen themselves and use resources that they have and sometimes teach you a little bit ...
>
> Becker et al. (2004, p. 336)

It is interesting to note that the advocates themselves were local women and they believed that the process of being advocates and working with local women empowered both participants.

In the UK, there are various buddying projects or projects where local women are recruited as advocates to promote health in their local community. There is potential for many of the projects to work in a similar way to the MOMobile scheme, although there has been little research into the women's experience of being involved in such projects. A research project has been evaluated that offered social support in pregnancy to a group of women who had given birth to a low-birthweight baby in a previous pregnancy (Oakley et al. 1996). Social support was given by research midwives, in addition to the usual midwifery care. The support took the form of home visits, when the research midwife provided a listening ear for the women. The research midwife was also available for 24-hour contact by the women. The physical and psychosocial outcomes for the group of women who were given extra support were better at 6 weeks, 1 year and 7 years after the birth of the child. The results of the research project appear to confirm that social support by midwives does promote health. Although empowerment is not specifically discussed in Oakley et al.'s research, it is possible that the social support offered by the research midwives facilitated the empowerment of the women included in the study through the support by the midwives of the women in making decisions.

As illustrated empowerment is a major influence on the ability to make healthier choices. Midwives have the potential to help women (and their partners) empower themselves through both group work and individual encounters.

SUMMARY OF KEY POINTS

The factors that mediate women's ability to make healthier choices include:

- The impact of family and home life. Domestic responsibilities and expectations may limit a woman's ability to care for her own health.
- The influence of power and control may prevent women accessing facilities or making choices.
- Being poor will make it harder for women to afford healthier options and more difficult to access facilities. Poverty may also mean that a woman's priorities may be at odds with the priorities of the Government or health agencies.
- Women from black and ethnic minority groups will have both the mediating factors of all women plus the additional constraints arising from their situation in the UK.
- There are a number of possible ways forward for engaging women in health promotion and facilitating healthy choices. There is a need to:
  - examine the practical restrictions on women making healthier choices
  - foster an environment that helps women empower themselves to make healthier choices in their lives.

REFERENCES

Ali N, Burchett H (2004) *Experiences of maternity services, perspectives of Muslim women.* London: Maternity Alliance: available on line at www.maternityalliance.org.uk/documents/Muslimwomenreport.pdf (accessed June 2005).

Ball K, Crawford D, Warren N (2003) How feasible are healthy eating and physical activity for young women? *Public Health Nutrition* 7: 433–41.

Baum FE, Ziersch AM (2003) Social capital. *Journal of Epidemiology and Community Health* 57: 320–3.

Becker J, Kovach A, Gronseth D (2004) Individual empowerment: How community health workers operationalize self-determination, self-sufficiency, and decision-making abilities of low-income mothers. *Journal of Community Psychology* 32: 327–42.

Boothroyd L (2002) Domestic violence: implications for children. *MIDIRS Midwifery Digest* 12(suppl 2): S9–S11.

Currie D, Weisenberg S (2003) Promoting women's health-seeking behaviour: Research and the empowerment of women, *Health Care for Women International* 24: 880–99.

Department of Health (2003) *Tackling Health Inequalities: A programme for action.* London: Department of Health.

Fawcett Society (2005) *Women and Poverty* (available on line at www.fawcettsociety.org.uk accessed June 2005).

Gostling LB (2003) Blakenell teenage club. *MIDIRS Midwifery Digest* 13: 408–10.

Hunt S (2004a) Poverty, pregnancy and childbirth. *The Practising Midwife* 7: 12–16.

Hunt S (2004b) *Poverty, Pregnancy and the Healthcare Professional.* Edinburgh: Books for Midwives.

Joffe H (2002) Representations of health risks: what social psychology can offer health promotion. *Health Education Journal* 61: 153–65.

Lewis G (2002) Domestic violence: lessons from the 1997–1999 confidential enquiry into maternal deaths (CEMD). *MIDIRS Midwifery Digest* 12(suppl 2): S6–S8.

Lynch J, Due P, Muntaner C, Davey Smith G (2000) Social capital – Is it a good investment strategy for public health. *Journal of Epidemiology and Community Health* 54: 404–8.

Oakley A, Hickey D, Rajan L (1996) Social support in pregnancy: does it have long-term effects? *Journal of Reproductive and Infant Psychology* 14: 7–22.

Pearce A, Mayho P (2004) Provision of antenatal care during Ramadan. *British Journal of Midwifery* 12: 750–2.

Peterson A, Hughey J (2004) Social cohesion and intrapersonal empowerment: gender as moderator. *Health Action Research* 19: 533–42.

Portela A, Santarelli C (2003) Empowerment of women, men, families and communities: true partnership for improving maternal and newborn health. *British Medical Bulletin* 67: 59–72.

Rosenblatt G, Rake K (2003) *Gender and Poverty.* London: Fawcett Society.

Rowe R, Garcia J (2003) Social class, ethnicity and attendance for antenatal care in the United Kingdom: a systematic review. *Journal of Public Health Medicine* 25: 113–19.

Royal College of Midwives (2004) *Making Maternity Services Work for Black and Ethnic Minority Women: A resource guide for midwives.* London: RCM.

Tones K (1991) Health promotion, empowerment and the psychology of control. *Journal of International Health Education* 29: 17–26.

Whitehead D, Russell G (2004) How effective are health education programmes – resistance, reaction, rationality and risk? Recommendations for effective practice. *International Journal of Nursing Studies* 41: 163–72.

Wurst JW, Merritt-Gray M, Berman H, Ford-Gilboe M (2002) Illuminating social determinants of women's health using grounded theory. *Health Care for Women International* 23: 794–808.

Wynn SW, Wynn AH, Doyle W (1994) The association of maternal social class with maternal diet and dimensions of babies in a population of London women. *Nutrition and Health* 9: 303–15.

4 USING HEALTH PROMOTION MODELS AND APPROACHES IN MIDWIFERY

JAN BOWDEN

Health promotion is itself a contested field of study, partly because it is a very broad field of action, incorporating many professions such as medicine, public health, education and midwifery, to name but a few, and because its focus has changed over time. With its wide scope and the multitude of outside influences affecting health, the development of approaches and models in health promotion has become a necessity. Theoretical and practical models and approaches have been used in disciplines such as science, medicine and nursing for some time. Within midwifery their development and use has not been as rapid partly as a result of the claim that the unique and individual situations of pregnancy and childbirth do not lend themselves to categorization of women, their families or their needs. Midwives' resistance may also be the result of our belief in our own autonomy as practitioners and in a more holistic approach to care. Most models used within midwifery have been adapted from nursing and medicine, which historically have illness as a starting point. However, if midwifery is to be viewed as a health-promoting activity, it may be that the health promotion models and approaches available can enhance the way that midwives deliver care. By the development of agreed research-based frameworks that have developed from a health stance, rather than an illness one, good practice may be standardized and prevent the labelling of women and their families. Within this chapter terms of reference are defined, and the approaches and models developed by Ewles and Simnett (2003), Downie et al. (1996) and Taylor (1990) explored and applied to health promotion within midwifery practice.

DEFINING TERMS

On scrutinizing the available literature from various disciplines that use models, it soon becomes very apparent that many terms of reference are used loosely and interchangeably. Examples of such terms are models, theories, conceptual frameworks, approaches, paradigms, taxonomies and ideologies. A brief glossary of these terms in relation to health promotion is provided here to avoid confusion. The terms 'model' and 'approach' are used throughout this chapter, unless an original author refers to his or her ideas by a different term.

Model

This is a single physical representation of a set of ideas, often diagrammatic, that provides assistance for our thinking and understanding of the underlying philosophical issues of both theory and practice. It attempts to be objective. Within disciplines such as health promotion, science and medicine models are used equally in reference to theory and/or philosophy (Crafter 1997, Seedhouse 2003), although in midwifery the term has been adopted a great deal, but not exclusively, to refer to the aspects of care given to women. Models give shape and in some way must either conform to a pattern, impose a pattern or reveal a pattern (Seedhouse 2003).

Theory

This is an organized or integrated set of propositions, which may or may not have been tested for its validity in relation to other theories put forward to explain the same situation. Different theories for the same situation may be equally valid, because the experience and 'truth' of one person may be different from those of another. A theory tends to be more subjective than a model. However, a model can be developed as a concrete representation of a tested theory (Crafter 1997, Seedhouse 2003).

Conceptual framework

This is a theoretical structure, under which ideas are formulated. It is more simplistic than a model and emanates from an individual's own early development of ideas, and may later develop into theories (Crafter 1997).

Approach

This literally implies a means of reaching a destination. Most authors refer to a set of approaches that attempt to encapsulate different ways of reaching the same objective, in this case delivering health promotion. An approach tends to be applicable to the philosophy as well as the practice of delivering care. Within health promotion the term is favoured by pragmatic practitioners, who focus on practicalities, and eclectic practitioners, who mix ideas arbitrarily, selecting and combining philosophies from various sources; it is tentative in its nature (Bunton and Macdonald 1992, Seedhouse 2003).

Paradigm

This is a wider concept than a theory. It constitutes an agreed way of looking at and interpreting a particular field of study or the world. It is used to predict the course of further investigation. It is an inherent part of a paradigm that the ideas are shown side by side, so that they can be compared and contrasted – hence the term 'paradigm map' (Bunton and Macdonald 1992).

Taxonomy

This is a categorical classification of elements into different groups or species, e.g. Bradshaw's classifications of needs (Bradshaw 1972, Seedhouse 2003).

Ideology

This is the study of ideas and is central to any discussion around models. It has a value system that fashions people's acuity of the human condition, human nature and society. This acuity engenders commitment to a particular course of action (or inaction). Therefore, ideology determines not only the model of health promotion to be used but also whether any intervention to promote health is desirable, worthwhile or even ethical (Seedhouse 2003).

WHY USE MODELS AND APPROACHES IN HEALTH PROMOTION?

Health promotion as identified earlier in Chapter 2 can be defined in many varied ways. There is no straightforward unity about the ideas that underpin health promotion and in particular the ideas that attempt to define what the principal health promotion goals should be. It is clear that health promotion is neither neutral nor value free, nor can it be, and its main protagonists have very different thoughts about priorities and strategies that reflect their own underlying values (Cribb and Duncan 2002).

This is the same for those who promote health. They will all have their own ideas based on their values and beliefs about health promotion and how it should be undertaken. These ideas, values and beliefs develop with time and experience. Their importance becomes apparent when working in a team or partnership where values are shared and made explicit, so that the health promoters can work towards the same goals. Thus the recipients of that health promotion can be clear about the standards and outcomes to expect. The Sure-Start programme provides a good example of this in practice.

The development of unified models and approaches in health promotion and midwifery can therefore help us to communicate with each other more effectively and strengthen initiatives, which benefits everybody. The more sophisticated models and approaches will also allow for individual holistic expression for both the midwife and the woman being cared for.

APPLYING HEALTH PROMOTION MODELS AND APPROACHES TO MIDWIFERY CARE

There is a plethora of models and approaches currently used within health promotion. This is perhaps testimony to the speed with which health promotion philosophy is advancing, and the need for theorists to develop their own framework to understand and explain, in as simple terms as possible, the relationship between the theory and the practice of health promotion. Some would argue that it identifies the status of health promotion as a profession and a field of study that is a relatively 'new kid on the block' (Cribb and Duncan 1999). Others have stated that this explosion of models and approaches is the result of the terrain of health promotion being strikingly large, loosely defined and continuously developing (Katz and Peberdy 2001). Some models and approaches are better known than others, often because they are more frequently quoted and used in the literature. The few explored here are chosen because they are frequently used within health promotion and midwifery literature, are relatively simple, can be easily applied to midwifery practice and serve to demonstrate how different from each other models and approaches can be, despite having the same general purpose.

Ewles and Simnett, in 1985, developed a framework of five approaches to health promotion, which were further elaborated on in 1992 (Ewles and Simnett 1992). This is a very influential approach and provides a significant example of mapping health promotion practice. It provides some of the values implicit in these approaches and allows a health promoter, i.e. the midwife, to clarify their aims and values when using them. In developing this framework the authors commented:

> In our view there is no 'right' aim for health promotion, and no one right approach or set of activities. We need to work out for ourselves, which aim and which activities we use, in accordance with our own professional code of conduct (if there is one), our own carefully considered needs and our own assessment of our clients' needs.
>
> Ewles and Simnett (1992, p. 37)

The medical approach

The aim here is freedom from medically defined diseases, illnesses and disability. This approach involves active medical participation to prevent or improve ill-health. An element of paternalism (one person deciding what is best for another) is involved because compliance is necessary on the part of the client/patient. Physical well-being tends to be the marker used to judge the success of the medical approach, with minimal or no reference to the psychological, social or economic aspects of the cause and effect of disease. This approach values preventive medical procedures. There has been much debate in recent years on the role and place of the medical approach in normal childbirth, and generally speaking it is now rejected by midwives and the Government as unsuitable for women (Royal College of Midwives (RCM) 2000, Department of Health (DoH) 2001). However, this approach is still used within midwifery, e.g. the screening for syphilis at booking and routine urinalysis and blood pressure checks for eclampsia.

The behaviour change approach

Here the midwife attempts to change the individual attitudes and behaviours of a woman. By doing so the midwife encourages the woman to adopt a 'healthier lifestyle', e.g. eating the right foods, sensible alcohol intake and stopping smoking. Some argue that, although this is a prominent feature of current health promotion practice in the UK, there is still a rather paternalistic element to it (Bunton et al. 2000). Models of behaviour change are looked at in more detail in Chapter 6.

The educational approach

In its most traditional sense the aim of this approach is that the educationalist, i.e. the midwife, will give the facts and information, with as few personal values as possible. The recipient, i.e. the woman, of this information is trusted to use it in whatever way she chooses – to continue with or abandon attitudes and behaviours as she wishes. The educationalist's responsibility is to raise issues. However, today this approach is seen very much as a two-directional approach, in that the midwife will provide information about a health issue and a woman will ask for information. This exchange should not be undertaken in isolation but in an environment where the woman's values and attitudes can be explored to help in her decision-making process.

The client-centred approach

Here the woman herself decides what the issues are and sets the agenda. This is considered to be a 'bottom-up' rather than a 'top-down' approach in which those in power and authority set the agenda. The woman is seen as an equal and the knowledge and skills that she brings to the interaction are valued. The theme of self-empowerment is pivotal. Some aspects of antenatal care are amenable to this approach in that, while blood pressure readings and other physical observations will always be important, their interpretation will demand the expertise of the midwife. There should always be an interaction that revolves around the issues raised by the woman herself. Available data show this approach to be a successful one (Hooton 2000, McLoughlin 2000, Ewles and Simnett 2003).

The societal change approach

This is Ewles and Simnett's only approach that does not directly concern the individual. Society is seen as central to health in that changes need to be made on social and environmental fronts, making the 'healthier option' easier to achieve for most of the population. An example of this societal change within the UK can be seen in the current discussions about banning smoking in public areas. Democratic movement towards such political action is said to make the whole environment more health enhancing.

The approaches offered by Ewles and Simnett are not without their problems. They can be seen as rather idealistic and simple in their layout. They do not necessarily address the issue of values, attitudes and beliefs held by both the health promoter, in this case the midwife, and the woman and her family, which will have a significant impact on their use. The authors themselves have identified that these approaches are not perfect and need to be questioned and challenged 'as part of a healthy debate on the theory and practice of health promotion' (Ewles and Simnett 2003, p. 46). However, the delineation of the approaches is clearly very useful in developing health promotion theory, and helping midwives to understand these approaches as well as clarifying their aims and values when using them.

Reflection – 1

Reflect on your two most recent health promotion activities within your current area of practice, e.g. a one-to-one interaction with a client, a group education programme such as a breastfeeding workshop or a community activity within Sure Start. Try to use different health promotion activities.

Looking at the approaches of Ewles and Simnett identified above pinpoint what approach/approaches you used.

In earlier work by Tannahill (1985), developed further by Downie et al. in 1990, a modern approach to health promotion was identified. This approach addressed issues surrounding positive health, life skills, self-esteem, participation, and dimensions of health, choice and behaviour. The authors identified that:

> The modern approach uses a broad information base and sound educational principles, and recognizes the importance of the sociopolitical factors in health and health related behaviours. It is a participatory model.
>
> Downie et al. (1990, p. 48)

Downie et al. (1996) developed this further and endorsed a model of health promotion, which maps out the various possible domains of health promotion. Three areas were identified:

1. Health education
2. Health prevention
3. Health protection.

These three areas frequently overlap (as shown in Figure 4.1) and within these overlapping circles lie the seven possible domains into which health promotion activities may fall.

Health education

This is defined as 'all influences that collectively determine knowledge, belief and behaviour related to the promotion, maintenance and restoration of health in

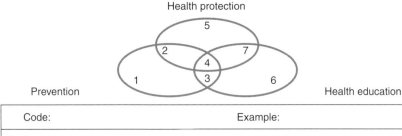

Code:	Example:
1. Prevention of disease, ill-health or abnormality	Preconception folic acid supplementation
2. Health education and prevention	'Stop smoking' campaigns
3. Prevention and health protection	Child vaccination programmes
4. Community development	Systematic antenatal care
5. Health education	Breastfeeding workshops
6. Health protection	Employment law for pregnant women
7. Health protection and health education	Campaigns by charity organizations to improve living and working conditions for pregnant women

FIGURE 4.1   *A model of health promotion. (Reproduced from Downie et al. 1996, with kind permission of Oxford University Press.)*

individuals and communities' (C Smith 1979; cited in Downie et al. 1996, p. 27). This includes incidental as well as intentional education, and Downie and his co-authors also acknowledge the two-way communication process of education, where teaching and learning can come from and to both the midwife and the woman.

Health prevention

This encompasses avoiding, or reducing, the risk of different forms of diseases, accidents and other forms of ill-health. It includes contraception, sexual health, and breast and cervical cancer screening. Downie et al. (1996, p. 51) went on to define the four aspects of prevention:

1. Prevention of the onset or first manifestation of a disease process or some other first occurrence through risk reduction.
2. Prevention of the progression of a disease process or other unwanted state through early detection.
3. Prevention of avoidable complications of an irreversible, manifest disease, or some other unwanted state.
4. Prevention of the recurrence of an illness or other unwanted phenomenon.

Health protection

This incorporates the environmental aspects safeguarding health by political, legislative and social control, which uses a number of mechanisms to achieve positive health by attempting to make the environment hazard free, such as regulation, policy and voluntary codes of practice.

In their approach Downie and his co-authors include both individual and community action in health promotion but exclude curative medicine. They acknowledge overlap in all of the three areas of health promotion that they describe, and see community action as the ultimate in health promotion because it broadly incorporates health education, prevention of disease and health protection. This model offers the health promoter many permutations; however, it does not make explicit the principal political or social values in each approach. Nor does it reveal the authors' preference as to the methods. Perhaps in not doing so the model offers the health promoter a greater autonomy than other models and approaches do, and make it more appealing to midwives who value their professional autonomy.

Ewles and Simnett's approach and that of Downie et al. are two of the most quoted in health promotion literature, and others commonly quoted use similar ideas. The two differ in that Ewles and Simnett (2003) construct their design from the perspective of the health promoter, whereas the Downie et al. (1996) perspective is that of health promotion outcomes. Nevertheless, the two approaches offer similarities. Ewles and Simnett's societal change approach and the element of community development in Downie et al.'s model have much in common. Both encourage community-based health care and each includes an educational approach. Downie et al. acknowledge all influences that lead to learning in clients and communities. However, Ewles and Simnett restrict their definition of education to that which allows individuals to exercise self-development by deciding, without undue pressure from outside, what the issues are and how to interpret them (Crafter 1997).

There are wide differences as well as similarities in the two approaches. Downie et al. do not include a medical approach in the curative sense (although they do acknowledge preventive medicine) and their model is distinct from that of Ewles and Simnett in this respect. The client-centred and behaviour change approaches of Ewles and Simnett find no reflection in Downie et al.'s model, the latter not suggesting how the outcomes of education, prevention and protection are reached. The major criticism of Ewles and Simnett's approach must be that, in describing from the perspective of the health promoter, it does not attend to possible outcomes of health promotion. Although the main criticism of Downie et al. must be that, in attending to outcomes, or products of health promotion, the process by which success is measured is missing (Crafter 1997).

Taylor (1990) provides a more sociological approach to what she refers to as health education, although on examining the breadth of her perspectives in today's terms she could be said to be referring to health promotion. Her ideas take the form of a paradigm map as shown in Figure 4.2.

Radical humanism

The perspective of radical humanism is that of self-development, particularly through personal growth, but with outreaching effects for community development. Removal from social regulation as far as possible is necessary and in some cases health professionals may be seen as social regulators, in that they are required to work strictly to rules and laws. A group of breastfeeding mothers running their own support group could be considered an example of the radical humanist approach.

Radical structuralism

Similar to radical humanism, radical structuralism is about moving towards change in the organization of society, and indeed is more concerned with changing society to remove barriers to health than changing the individual. Radical structuralism may be exemplified by a nationwide campaign to encourage breastfeeding, including legislation to improve maternity leave, an advertising campaign among the public to improve attitudes towards breastfeeding and the provision of widespread facilities for breastfeeding mothers.

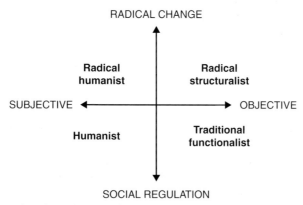

FIGURE 4.2 *Perspectives of health education. (Reproduced from Taylor 1990, with kind permission of the Health Education Journal.)*

Traditional functionalism

The traditional functionalist may be seen as the professional who possesses the expertise that is passed on to the layperson, who can then progress to healthier behaviours. An example of traditional functionalism is the existence of antenatal classes aimed at promoting breastfeeding.

Humanism

The humanist is concerned with personal autonomy and empowering individuals through life skills development. A network of NHS breastfeeding counsellors illustrates the humanist quarter of the map.

Elements of other approaches can be seen in Taylor's ideas, e.g. the traditional functionalist perspective reflects elements of Ewles and Simnett's medical and behaviour change approaches, and radical structuralism has some common ground with Downie et al.'s health protection approach, in that it is concerned with political and societal changes to improve the health of the public. However, overall, the sociological background to Taylor's paradigm is so different from the more clinical frameworks set by Ewles and Simnett and Downie et al. as to make these three systems impossible to compare (Crafter 1997).

Similar themes run through many of the health promotion models and approaches used currently in practice but each has a different area of emphasis. Central to contemporary health promotion is whether action should primarily focus on educating individuals and small groups, or on restructuring society to benefit everybody's health. This unresolved debate is reflected in the various models and approaches. The problem with focusing on individual responsibility in health is that the collective responsibility of health can be lost, leading to the scapegoating of sick or socially excluded individuals such as teenage pregnant women and pregnant women who experience domestic violence, when it would be better to improve health for a greater number of people by addressing change and health inequalities in society (Crafter 1997, Dufty 2005). Creators of models and approaches must aim as far as possible to design very broad frameworks that acknowledge the political dimension of health-care administration, as well as recognize the day-to-day practicalities for health promoters working with individuals in the community.

USING HEALTH PROMOTION MODELS AND APPROACHES IN MIDWIFERY

Although examples of situations common to midwives have been chosen in this chapter in relation to a few models and approaches, it remains to demonstrate how, overall, midwives can use these approaches to understand individuals' different outlooks, and work towards a minimum standard of high-quality practice and common goals. Crafter (1997, pp. 73–5) took smoking cessation as an example of how these models and approaches could be applied to midwifery. She used as an example the midwives of Newplace Hospital, who note high cigarette smoking rates among pregnant women and wish to incorporate in their service a plan to reduce these rates, and to tackle the related problems of longer term ill health and prematurity in the babies.

In formulating their action plan, Crafter's group base their strategy on the approaches of Ewles and Simnett to take account of as many tactics as possible (their interpretation of its application may be as follows).

The medical approach

Activities under this heading may include the following:

- Offering women who smoke examination of cardiac and respiratory function at various stages throughout pregnancy to check for and treat smoking-induced disease
- Offering advice to stop smoking
- Provision of neonatal intensive and special care facilities
- Collection and collation of national and local smoking statistics, against which Newplace Hospital can check its progress.

The behaviour change approach

Activities include setting up smoking cessation classes and inviting smokers to attend. Incentives for attendance such as free baby supplies may be applied. The methods used to achieve the stated aim of reducing smoking rates is that of persuasion, and facts and figures relating to the dangers of cigarette smoking are given to fortify women in their decision to try to stop smoking plus ongoing support by the midwife to help maintain the change. However, problems arise in assessing women's smoking habits and the provision of midwives to provide the continuous help and support needed.

The educational approach

The midwives run into problems here because, in reality, they have set their aim to reduce smoking in childbearing women so they cannot exclude this personal value – that smoking is harmful and therefore bad – from their approach to smoking in pregnancy. A true educational approach is therefore not possible, because the women are being given value-laden facts and information, and not being supported in their own decision as to whether or not to continue or cut down on their smoking habit. However, while acknowledging this problem, the midwives could adapt Ewles and Simnett's approaches to suit their own ends better, and concentrate on 'an awareness approach' (rather than tackling smoking cessation) with women and their partners in classes or during antenatal appointments. Posters and leaflets about smoking may be displayed around the hospital. Women and couples could be encouraged to explore their own attitudes, values and reasons for smoking. Staff training and support will also be necessary, so staff are not drawn into coercing or judging women who choose to exercise their free will when this is in conflict with the hospital's objective to reduce smoking levels. (Smoking cessation is discussed in Chapter 12.)

The client-centred approach

Again, the midwives will find themselves running into a moral minefield because they have already set the agenda and so the 'clients' are excluded from deciding what the issues are. A further adaptation of Ewles and Simnett's ideas is necessary if the midwives wish to involve people from the local community, which would be sensible. They may decide to call this a 'community involvement approach'. Activities may include contacting the Maternity Alliance, the local maternity services liaison committee and any other interested groups or individuals, particularly women smokers of reproductive age, who would be invited to comment on what initiatives they would like the hospital to institute in order to reduce the medical and social problems induced by smoking. However, asking such groups for their input after deciding to reduce maternal smoking in the area may well induce some heated argument about human rights (including fetal rights) and the role of the health services in prescribing 'good' behaviour to a population. A suggestion box in the hospital, for women to leave anonymous ideas, may get some interesting suggestions from individuals, but again this is not truly client centred, just giving token support to the idea of client involvement.

A truly client-centred approach could occur only if a midwife had no pre-conceived ideas about what smoking women should think and do when pregnancy is confirmed, and encouraged such women to voice their feelings about smoking. However, when such a woman comes forward for antenatal care, and asks for help to reduce or stop her habit, the midwife can use strategies to empower the woman to find the motivation and means to fulfil her wishes. This may include giving the woman information about smoking cessation groups in the area. In this context, the client-centred approach would be little different from the educational approach.

The societal change approach

Activities here are directed at the general hospital environment, and the midwives, together with other members of staff, are likely to designate all or most of it a no smoking area. However, decisions need to be made about how to deal with heavily addicted smokers in the hospital who may smoke in unsuitable areas if driven to secrecy and may dispose of butts in dangerous places. A smoking cessation course may be offered to members of staff, free of charge and possibly in hospital time. Problems may arise with members of staff who are happy smokers and do not wish to stop their habit or, more difficult still, do not agree with, or wish to take part in, the hospital drive to reduce smoking among its users.

In considering such an activity as reducing smoking rates, it can be seen that planning the intervention using health promotion models and approaches adds many dimensions to the activity, and gives structure to its implementation. However, it also throws up many dilemmas, of a practical and ethical nature, that need to be resolved as the activity progresses (or, better still, before it has started) (Cribb and Duncan 2002). Some of these problems take a considerable time to resolve, and universal consensus as to how to go about the seemingly altruistic and admirable aim of reducing smoking rates and improving maternal and infant health may seem insurmountable. Without strong-minded and versatile leaders and players, this probably demonstrates as well as any argument why change is so difficult to implement in hospitals and health promotion programmes!

SUMMARY OF KEY POINTS

- Health promotion models and approaches provide a spur to examine and re-examine practice and its underlying assumptions.
- Terms such as model, theory, conceptual framework, approach and paradigm are sometimes used interchangeably in the health promotion literature.
- The plethora of models and approaches currently in use is often criticized for being perplexing and ineffectual.
- Effective models and approaches serve to state the relationship between the theory and practice of health promotion There is a moral requirement for the midwife to be clear about this relationship because, where an attempt is made to change people's behaviour, as often happens, the ethical dimensions of such professional practice are immense.
- Models and approaches in health promotion can help us to communicate more effectively by concentrating discussion on shared values and beliefs relevant to professional practice, and putting these into a framework that explicitly states acceptable standards of practice, to both the midwife and the women in her care.
- The application of health promotion models and approaches to some aspects of midwifery practice can offer a means by which agreed evidence-based frameworks standardize good practice.
- The study and application of various health promotion models and approaches to midwifery practice can help us to understand different outlooks and develop innovative strategies suited to particular communities.

REFERENCES

Bradshaw J (1972) The concept of social need. *New Society* **52**: 141–50.

Bunton R, Baldwi S, Flynn D, Whitelaw S (2000) The 'stages of change' model in health promotion. Science and ideology. *Critical Public Health* **10**: 55–70.

Bunton R, Macdonald G (eds) (1992) *Health Promotion: Disciplines and diversity*. London: Routledge.

Crafter H (ed.) (1997) Using health promotion models and approaches in midwifery. In: *Health Promotion in Midwifery Principles and Practice*. London: Arnold.

Cribb A, Duncan P (1999) Making a profession of health promotion? Grounds for trust and health promotion ethics. *International Journal of Health Promotion and Health Education* **37**: 129–34.

Cribb A, Duncan P (2002) *Health Promotion and Professional Ethics*. London: Blackwell Science.

Department of Health (2001) *Making a Difference: The nursing, midwifery and health visiting contribution: The Midwifery Action Plan*. London: The Stationery Office.

Downie RS, Fyfe C, Tannahill A (1990) *Health Promotion Models and Values*. Oxford: Oxford Medical Publications.

Downie RS, Tannahill C, Tannahill A (1996) *Health Promotion, Models and Values*, 2nd edn. Oxford: Oxford University Press.

Dufty J (2005) They have only themselves to blame … . Understanding the political, psychosocial and environmental drivers that power the trend for unhealthy lifestyles behaviours in deprived communities. *MIDIRS Midwifery Digest* **15**: 115–20.

Ewles L, Simnett I (1992) *Promoting Health: A practical guide*, 2nd edn. London: Baillière Tindall.

Ewles L, Simnett I (2003) *Promoting Health: A practical guide*, 5th edn. London: Scutari Press.

Hooton S (2000) Promoting child and family health through empowerment. In: Kerr J (ed.), *Community Health Promotion Challenges for Practice*. London: Baillière Tindall, pp. 101–123.

Katz J, Peberdy A (2001) *Promoting Health: Knowledge and practice*, 2nd edn. London: Macmillan.

McLoughlin A (2000) Empowerment and childbirth. In: Kerr J (ed.), *Community Health Promotion Challenges for Practice*. London: Baillière Tindall, pp. 65–81.

Royal College of Midwives (2000) *The Midwife's Role in Public Health: Position Paper No. 24*. London: RCM.

Seedhouse D (2003) *Health Promotion Philosophy, Prejudice and Practice*, 2nd edn. Chichester: John Wiley & Sons Ltd.

Tannahill A (1985) What is health promotion? *Health Education Journal* **44**: 167–8.

Taylor V (1990) Health education – a theoretical mapping. *Health Education Journal* **49**: 13–14.

FURTHER READING

Cribb A, Duncan P (2002) *Health Promotion and Professional Ethics*. London: Blackwell Science.

Hooton S (2000) Promoting child and family health through empowerment. In: Kerr J (ed.), *Community Health Promotion Challenges for Practice*. London: Baillière Tindall.

McLoughlin A (2000) Empowerment and childbirth. In: Kerr J (ed.), *Community Health Promotion Challenges for Practice*. London: Baillière Tindall.

Seedhouse D (2003) *Health Promotion Philosophy, Prejudice and Practice*, 2nd edn. Chichester: John Wiley & Sons Ltd.

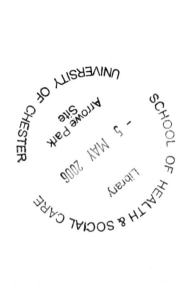

5 EVALUATING HEALTH PROMOTION ACTIVITIES

JAN BOWDEN

Currently within the National Health Service (NHS) there is a drive to evaluate all aspects of health to ensure that all practices, including health promotion, are evidence based. Bearing in mind the 'new kid on the block' status of health promotion as a profession and field of study, there is added impetus for evaluation to take place to prove its worth. Evaluation in health promotion is not as straightforward as it seems. The waters are muddied by a combination of factors such as: the long timescale of projects, the many kinds of activities involved in a health-promoting project and the many stakeholders working in partnership, all of whom may have their own different objectives. The use of the randomized control trial (RCT) as the gold standard for evaluation in the health arena also complicates the evaluation of health promotion that does not fit neatly into the RCT model. This chapter, with relevant research evidence, examines what is meant by evaluation, and for whom and why it is undertaken, as well as addressing the process and challenges of evaluating a health promotion activity.

WHAT IS EVALUATION AND WHY DO IT?

The *Oxford Concise Dictionary of Current English* (Allen 1993) defines evaluation as 'the process of assessing and appraising'. It is a process in which we are involved daily both as a professional and as an individual. If evaluation is about assessing or appraising the worth of an activity, then we are involved in that process whenever we reflect upon our actions and either alter them or continue them (Katz and Perberdy 2001).

Within health promotion evaluation occurs from practice and is aimed explicitly at reflecting on and shaping practice. Tones and Tilford (1994, p. 49) stated that:

> Evaluation is concerned with assessing an activity against values and goals in such a way that results can contribute to future decision-making and/or policy ...

Evaluation is guided by two essential principles: identifying and ranking the criteria (value and aims), and gathering data and information that will make it possible to measure to what degree these criteria are being or have been met. There are different criteria that can be used when a health promotion activity is being judged on its worth.

Effectiveness

This is concerned with whether the activity has accomplished what it set out to do and to what extent the aims and objectives were met. It is essential to realize that, although in practice the terms 'aims' and 'objectives' are used interchangeably, it is vital to know that there is an important difference. Aims tend to be general and may be divided into particular objectives. Objectives contribute to the aims and are the 'nuts and bolts' of the planned project. Both are vital to the evaluation process. Poor identification of aims and objectives within a project will make evaluation impossible (Katz and Perberdy 2001, Rootman et al. 2001).

Appropriateness

This is assessing the relevance of the intervention to needs. The perception of needs differs depending on who is defining them: the individual/group requiring the health promotion project or the health professionals who develop the project (Bradshaw 1972, Ewles and Simnett 2003).

Acceptability

This assesses whether the project is being carried out in a sensitive way. This is sometimes overlooked and a health promotion project may have ethical and moral values that affect its use either in the community for which it was intended or when the project is used in another community, e.g. a considerable quantity of the initial UK health education information on HIV and AIDS in the 1980s portrayed the genesis of HIV firmly in Africa and the developing world. This promoted racist typecasting and caused immense distress to many black and ethnic minority communities (Katz and Perberdy 2001).

Efficiency

This assesses whether time, money and resources are well spent given the benefits of the project. In recent years the ratio of costs to benefits has increased in import-ance. Assessment needs to involve *cost-effectiveness analysis* (the comparison of the financial costs of similar projects) and *cost–benefits analysis* (the comparison of the cost of the project with the financial benefits resulting from achieving the goal) (Tones and Tilford 1994, Katz and Perberdy 2001).

Equity

This assesses how accessible a project is. It goes beyond the identification of the num-bers that a project reaches. Equity evaluates the social composition that the project has reached. Some have stated that health promotion should go all out for equity over equality by not always aiming for equal access but intentionally aiming at those in socially excluded groups (Catford 1993, Katz and Perberdy 2001, Rootman et al. 2001).

For evaluation to be successful it must be built into the health promotion project from the planning stage and be ongoing and explicit at all times during the lifetime of that project. The complexity comes when this process of evaluation becomes formalized and with it the potential for it to become 'public', in that it is open to inspection and criticism by others (Katz and Perberdy 2001, Ewles and Simnett 2003). A further difficulty arises in the fact that health promotion can be an ambiguous affair with no assurances that specific effects will follow particular inputs (Naidoo and Wills 2000).

Activity – 1

Think about why evaluation is an essential element of health promotion. Compare your thoughts with Figure 5.1.

So why evaluate? Evaluation provides the best sort of feedback on which to develop health promotion projects. If the responses of users of the service are considered as essential to achieving aims, their opinions and comments can serve only to help the health promoter – in this case the midwife – to develop health promotional work. In recent years there has been much debate about the reasons for the development of this evaluation culture within health. Some argue that it has a political and ideological function to legitimize the actions of governments (Naidoo and Wills 2000, Katz and Perberdy 2001). Irrespective of this debate there are many possible reasons about why evaluation is required and needed within health promotion and Figure 5.1 identifies possible reasons for evaluation. It is important to stress that

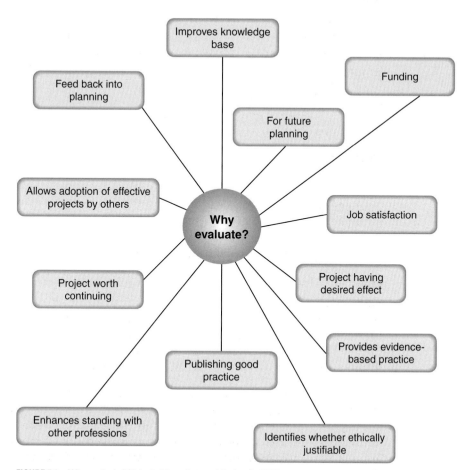

FIGURE 5.1 *Why evaluate? (Adapted from Katz and Perberdy 2001)*

Figure 5.1 offers only some suggestions and is not finite and you may well be able to add more.

WHO IS IT FOR AND WHO SHOULD DO IT?

Evaluation is undertaken for many reasons, as seen in Figure 5.1, and from this it can be argued that there are several groups and individuals for whom evaluation is beneficial and necessary. Ideally evaluation is best undertaken in a way that will allow each of the different stakeholders involved in the project to see if their aims and objectives have been met. Those who are funding the project may want the evaluation to show the efficiency of the project and its cost-effectiveness. This would allow them to see if their money had been well spent during the course of the project and to assess whether it requires continued longer-term funding or a possible reduction in funding. The health promoters may want the evaluation to show that their objectives have been met and that the project identified an acceptable way of working with the clients/community groups. They may also use it to 'push' for the project to be rolled out to other communities within their trust areas. Health promotion managers may look upon the evaluation as a way to assess performance and productivity. The users may use the evaluation as a way of signifying some degree of control over health-related aspects of their lives and of gaining ownership of the project. Finally, the Government (or local government even) may use the evaluation to justify their policies and strategies for health (Naidoo and Wills 2000, Katz and Perberdy 2001).

After identifying for whom the evaluation may be required, one must now examine who is going to evaluate the project, because after identifying the importance of evaluation the choice of who is going to undertake it is vital. Most evaluation is undertaken internally and this is an accepted practice within health promotion. Internal evaluation allows for a more continuous process of evaluation to take place, because those evaluating are always available. It is seen as non-threatening so all stakeholders are more able to be truthful about the project. However, internal evaluation does have its problems. Evidence suggests that it does not always fully evaluate a project as a result of issues such as lack of time and inexperience in evaluation, which are less likely to be made 'public', i.e. open for inspection (Nutbeam 1998, Rootman et al. 2001). This means that poor projects are not always properly evaluated, which in turn means that a valuable learning experience is lost. Equally, good projects are not brought to closer or wider attention and the knowledge and practice base are not enhanced (Nutbeam 1998, Rootman et al. 2001). External evaluation is seen as more beneficial because it tends to be carried out by individuals who are well versed in the practice of evaluation. It also tends to be more thorough with all stakeholders being asked their viewpoints. However, it is likely to suffer from issues associated with the evaluators being seen as outsiders and the stakeholders perhaps putting on a 'united front', and may also be more expensive (Rootman et al. 2001, Valente 2002). Table 5.1 attempts to identify more of the advantages and disadvantages of internal and external evaluation. Irrespective of whether evaluation is internal or external, 'a warts and all' approach to evaluation must be considered within health promotion to gain vital learning experience from both good and not so good health promotion projects (McQueen 2002, Potvin et al. 2005).

TABLE 5.1 *Advantages and disadvantages of internal and external evaluation*

Internal evaluation	External evaluation
Knows background to project	Fresh viewpoint
Known and therefore accepted more readily	More objective
Easier to establish networks of communication	No allegiance to the project
Knowledge about the community the project is intended for and therefore aware of any issues	Unbiased attitude
Usually has some idea of weakness and strengths of the project	More likely to have research expertise
Financially beneficial as usually cheaper	More likely to have experience in evaluation
Too involved in the project	More likely to be made 'public'
Biased towards proving the success of the project	More likely to be thorough
Less likely to have research expertise	More likely to access the views of all the stakeholders including the users
Less likely to have experience in evaluation	More likely that all the stakeholders will receive the evaluation report
Time constraints prevent a thorough evaluation	Less accepted as seen as outsiders
Users may not be so honest with their evaluation because they know the evaluator	Networks of communication more difficult to establish
	More expensive than internal evaluation
	Lacks knowledge about the project and the community for whom it is intended
	Stakeholders may portray a 'united front' for the external evaluation

Adapted from Naidoo and Wills (2000) and Katz and Perberdy (2001).

USER EVALUATION

Health promotion is a complex process of intervention in an individual's or community's life at varying levels. Therefore, it must be justified and evaluated by the individual and community at whom it is aimed, allowing them to have their story heard. In recent years the Department of Health (DoH), the NHS Executive, and various research charities and funding bodies have emphasized the importance of user involvement (DoH 1999, 2000). However, have users been included merely to satisfy regulations from the DoH and other funding bodies or is there a genuine conviction that their views are valuable to the evaluation process? By being used actively within the evaluation process users will, similar to external evaluation, provide a fresh perspective on the health promotion project. It will provide ownership of the project and allow the user to shape and guide the project and alter its organizational culture (Entwistle et al. 1998, Trivedi and Wykes 2002). Active user evaluation will add value and legitimacy to the project and potentially generate knowledge that could increase its significance and acceptance (Entwistle et al. 1998, Beresford 2002).

If users are given only a token involvement in evaluation, their role will be different and it is less likely that their story will be fully told, leaving them frustrated at not being heard or being allowed to be heard. Ownership will be with the 'experts' and the organizational culture will remain firmly within a professional remit. This, in turn, may affect the validity of the project and its sustainability within the community at which it is aimed (Entwistle et al. 1998, Beresford 2002). To facilitate user involvement within the project and the evaluation process, consideration must be given to include users from the birth of the project and for them to undertake some training about their role within the project. Training for professionals must also be considered to allow them to understand lay perspectives and to work effectively with users in different situations (Entwistle et al. 1998, Trivedi and Wykes 2002).

HOW BEST TO EVALUATE SUCCESS?

As already identified, evaluation in health promotion helps build a foundation of research and enquiry that allows health promotion to demonstrate its success in meeting its aims and objectives. It allows effective health promotion practices to be identified and used by others. It also allows these health promotion practices to be further developed and enhanced. This evidence-based practice, which is defined as 'the conscientious, explicit and judicious use of current evidence in making decisions about the care of the individual patient' (Sackett et al. 1996, p. 42), has already been established in other areas of health such as midwifery, nursing and medicine, where randomized controlled trials (RCTs) have been used to identify the most effective treatment and care for the most number of people. However, the RCT is not a tool that can be neatly fitted into health promotion. It is problematic for several reasons:

- It is impossible to isolate the effect of a health promotion project owing to the multiplicity of factors involved.
- A project's success is in some part due to its spread to other groups beyond the target group.
- The length of time that many projects take.
- The number of stakeholders, each with their own aims, objectives and viewpoints which they want to achieve.
- The awareness of health promoters of the social and cultural context in which they carry out their work.

Health promotion therefore suits a more social science approach to evaluation. It would allow for a much broader use of different methodologies from both the quantitative and the qualitative approaches. The different stakeholders and their individual viewpoints would also be taken into account, making the evaluation pluralistic (Means and Smith 1988, Naidoo and Wills 2000). This of course may lead to the criticisms that there is a lack methodological rigor and that the pluralistic approach is complex and lacks clarity (Hepworth 1997, Rootman et al. 2001).

The difficulties in evaluating health promotion led Nutbeam and his colleagues to develop a six-stage model demonstrating an evaluation hierarchy which identifies how best to evaluate success in health promotion (Nutbeam et al. 1990, 1993, Nutbeam 1996, 1998). There are six stages:

1. Problem definition

This draws upon the data used to identify the health issue on which the health promotion project has to improve. This information relies on epidemiological data and needs appraisal to define the problem, the factors influential to the problem and the scope for change.

2. Solution generation

This explores the behavioural and social research to expand the knowledge of the targeted population and the breadth of personal, social, environmental and organizational features that may need to be adapted to form the basis for the project. It will also help to explain and predict change in those features as well as clarifying the potential content and approaches for the intervention. Stages 1 and 2 will help with the success and sustainability of the project developed.

3. Testing innovation

This is where the process, impact and outcome of the project are judged.

Process evaluation

This is concerned with the assessment of the implementation and maintenance of the activity. Sometimes called formative or illuminative evaluation, it also focuses on the acuity and responses of the participants to the health promotion project (Katz and Perberdy 2001). Moreover, it attempts to identify the factors that have hindered the project, as well as ascertain those that have supported it. Process evaluation is a useful mechanism to gauge the acceptability as well as the appropriateness and equity of a health promotion project. Interviews, diaries and observations are some of the 'soft' qualitative methods that process evaluation uses to gain details about a project. However, the use of qualitative evaluation methods is often dismissed because they lack the 'scientific' credibility of the 'hard' quantitative evaluation approaches and are often criticized for being unrepresentative (Naidoo and Wills 2000, Rootman et al. 2001).

Impact evaluation

The evaluation of a health promotion project is usually concerned with identification of the effects of the project. The easiest and therefore the most popular way to undertake this is by assessing the immediate effect that the activity has on the recipients' knowledge, attitudes, behaviour and short-term health change (Naidoo and Wills 2000). The midwife collects these data at the time of finishing the activity or shortly after. Data collected tend to be of a quantitative nature, with all the usual criticisms.

Outcome evaluation

This can seen as the real test of whether the initial aims and objectives have been achieved. Outcome evaluation is more difficult and complex because it looks at evaluating the longer-term impact of the health promotion project. This may mean the midwife having to contact clients a year after the project has finished. However, despite these issues outcome evaluation tends to be much preferred. It attempts to evaluate changes that have stood the test of time. This evaluation often uses control groups and data that are expressed numerically, which increases its credibility because it is seen as more accurate and more like the quantitative approach (Naidoo and Wills 2000, Rootman et al. 2001).

4. Intervention demonstration

This stage changes emphasis slightly from the assessment of process, impact and outcome, and looks more closely at the conditions for success or lack of success. It will assess the achievement of the project under ideal circumstances and then look at whether the desired outcomes of the project can be achieved in a more 'real' environment. This is particularly relevant to the communities that are targeted for the project, as well as the health promoters, because it looks at the achievability of the project in everyday life. It will also take into account the unpredictable facets of health promotion practice and identify what basics need to be in place for it to be a success.

5. Intervention dissemination

In this fifth stage the emphasis is further moved to look at ways in which successfully evaluated projects can be disseminated. This dissemination would advance evidence-based practice by investigating what others have done and, through use of their experiences, aid other health promotion projects. Understanding how individuals and communities adopt and maintain a healthier lifestyle and what support is needed to assist this, determining what basics need to be in place to facilitate the success of a project as well as highlighting what needs to be done, by whom, to what criterion and to what cost, would be some of the benefits of intervention dissemination. However, it is rarely undertaken.

6. Programme management

In this stage the evaluation tasks are directed totally towards the maintenance of the project. Evaluation will incorporate the monitoring of the project's delivery in relation to its optimal conditions for success and, of course, value for money. The project's sustainability and longevity will be continuously evaluated.

CHALLENGES TO EVALUATION IN HEALTH PROMOTION

There are several challenges for a midwife wishing to evaluate either the midwife's role within health promotion or a midwifery-based or midwifery-led health promotion project. Naidoo and Wills (2000) identified the following challenges that will be faced by the health professional – in this case the midwife – when involved in health promotion evaluation:

- What needs to be measured?
- Are the effects entirely the result of the health promotion project?
- When to evaluate?
- What signifies success in a project?
- Is the effort worth it?
- What ethical issues are related to evaluation?

What needs to be measured?

This is not as easy as it would seem. The essential tenet has to be measurement of the objectives decided on, which is undertaken in the planning stage of the health promotion project. This appears to be reasonably straightforward; however, on reviewing the literature, the midwife may find numerous published studies that breach this simple golden rule (Naidoo and Wills 2000, Seedhouse 2003). The biggest problem appears to be a lack of consensus between the stakeholders about the suitable measurements, e.g. trying to measure the involvement of a community in relation to breastfeeding or showing an increase in breastfeeding rates as a result of the development of breastfeeding workshops is not easy because of the other factors that may be involved, e.g. influence of peers, families and media.

Are the effects entirely the result of the health promotion project?

Health promotion is not a quick fix solution and because the situation varies constantly it can be very difficult to be confident that the results of a health promotion project are solely the result of the input of that project (Rootman et al. 2001). Health promotion is a long-term process and, during that period of time, health-related knowledge, attitudes and behaviours will have changed on the part of the health promoter and the targeted population. Society also constantly reacts to varying factors, so the success of a health promotion project may be caused more by societal change than the actual project (Naidoo and Wills 2000, Katz and Perberdy 2001, Potvin et al. 2005), e.g. the success of smoking cessation workshops for pregnant women who smoke may not be the result of to the workshops themselves so much as society's changing views on smoking. Also a project's success is in some part the result of its spread to other groups beyond the target population. It would be very difficult to prevent the health promotion project 'seeping out' beyond its targeted population (Naidoo and Wills 2000).

When to evaluate?

As a result of the process of health promotion, a health promotion project may have different outcomes at different times in the lifetime of the project. Timing is vital when evaluating the success of a health promotion project, e.g. a breastfeeding promotion project may have several outcomes:

- Improvement in women's knowledge of breastfeeding.
- Increase in numbers of women attending breastfeeding workshops.
- Increase in local (and perhaps national) media coverage on breastfeeding.
- Persuasion of local restaurants, cafes and shops to advertise that women may breastfeed within their environs.
- Encouragement of various organizations to adopt pro-breastfeeding measures, i.e. local employers.
- Reduction in the number of babies admitted to hospital with formula feed-related gastroenteritis.

(Adapted from Naidoo and Wills 2000.)

Each of these outcomes will need to be evaluated at different times to be able to prove the project's success or indeed identify its failure. However, there is no researched theory to assist with the solution to this timing issue and health promoters tend to work on their own previous experience or the experience of other projects as to when to evaluate, e.g. when working through the evaluation on the above-mentioned breastfeeding promotion project the midwife may consider the following: an immediate evaluation of the project to ascertain the success of the first outcome and an interim evaluation at 3–6 months to identify the outcomes regarding the numbers of women attending the breastfeeding workshops and the increase in media coverage. However, the remaining outcomes may need a much longer period of time to elapse before evaluation is possible – as long as 5 years. This raises the issue of whether the success of the project is the result of the project alone or of changes within the community or society.

What signifies success in a project?

Investigation of what others have done and the use of their experiences to aid other health promotion projects is one way of proving effectiveness. Effectiveness reviews assist health promotion in two ways: first by evaluating the quality of the research and second the quality of the health promotion project (Nutbeam 1998, Rootman et al. 2001). They also identify a means by which a foundation of knowledge is cultivated to pinpoint what the reasonable expectations of a successful project are. This in itself is problematical on several counts:

1. Health promotion is concerned with changing health knowledge, behaviours and attitudes on many different levels over a sometimes lengthy time period. It therefore requires a multi-pronged evaluation process that is fraught with difficulties.
2. The preferred 'gold standard' of an RCT does not fit well in health promotion where feelings, behaviours, attitudes and changes to these are not easily expressed numerically.
3. Effectiveness reviews are the least common health promotion research found in the health promotion literature, resulting partly from a lack of interest in this area of research and partly from the limited number of projects that have reached a stage of development that allows an effectiveness review to be undertaken (Nutbeam 1998).

Is it worth the effort?

Appraising the value or worth of one's work is an essential component of being a reflective practitioner. However, in light of all the difficulties that evaluation in health promotion faces, a decision to undertake a more formal evaluation of that work and making it 'public' is not so easy. The dilemmas of what to measure, how to measure, when to measure and what constitutes success are faced by all health promoters who undertake evaluation of their project. For a midwife measuring her own effectiveness in delivering a small-scale health-promoting project, reliability and validity are of little consequence. However, for larger project evaluation, these concepts must be addressed to make sure that the results obtained are not spurious. Provided that evaluation is built into the health promotion project from the planning stage and is ongoing and explicit at all times during the lifetime of that project, it is worth the effort. Providing the evaluation is explicated and fed back into the project, and to the stakeholders, it is worth it. It is not worth the effort if evaluation is seen as an 'add on' to the project buried under complicated and inappropriate evaluation tools and not fed back at all.

What ethical issues are related to evaluation?

The inconvenience of any evaluation should be considered and weighed up against the value of the information that it provides. Although *not* evaluating health promotional projects has major and obvious ethical dimensions, to evaluate must also be viewed in an ethical context. Downie et al. (1996) comment on the need to evaluate whether health promotional activities are ethically justified. There are a number of ethical issues here that deserve consideration. The first is whose interests does the evaluation serve? The politics of vested interests in choosing an evaluation technique and the issue of who receives the findings, and what they do with them, are very pertinent when evaluating a health promotion project. Evaluation can be time-consuming for recipients and frustrating if they do not see any change as a result of the comments that they have given. Although future recipients may benefit from previous evaluations if the information gained was made use of, they will not benefit if the evaluator has not done anything with the findings. This often happens if the evaluation gives information that is difficult to interpret because the aims of the project were not clearly thought out at the beginning. It also occurs when the evaluation gives such a wide range of feedback that it is impossible to decide whether the project has been effective, and where improvements could be made.

Given that an evaluation has been reasonably well carried out and conclusions drawn, decisions must be made about who holds responsibility for incorporating the findings in future practice. If the conclusions recommend the investment of further resources, it may be impossible for the non-budget-holding evaluator to act. Aims and objectives almost always include an element of behaviour change, which may cause personal discomfort and have an effect on the recipients' relationships with family and friends. The effect of education cannot be predicted and, as seen in the film *Educating Rita*, where Rita's new knowledge leaves her abandoned by her husband and old friends and feeling misunderstood by her family, it can be a double-edged sword (Crafter 1997).

SUMMARY OF KEY POINTS

- Currently, within the National Health Service (NHS), there is a drive to evaluate all aspects of health to ensure that all practices including health promotion are evidence based. Bearing in mind the 'new kid on the block' status of health promotion as a profession and a field of study, there is added impetus for evaluation to take place to prove its worth.
- Evaluation is formed of two essential parts: identifying and ranking the criteria (value and aims) and gathering data and information that will make it possible to measure to what degree these criteria are being or have been met.
- When judging the worth of a health promotion project, effectiveness, appropriateness, acceptability, efficiency and equity must be considered.
- Health promotion is concerned with changing health knowledge, behaviours and attitudes on many different levels over a sometimes lengthy time period. It therefore requires a multi-pronged evaluation process that is fraught with difficulties.
- The preferred 'gold standard' of RCT does not fit well in health promotion where feelings, behaviours, attitudes and changes to these are not easily expressed numerically.
- There are several challenges for a midwife wishing to evaluate either the midwife's role within health promotion or a midwifery-based or midwifery-led health promotion project. The biggest of these is the fact that 'evaluation within health promotion is a difficult enterprise which is often poorly done' (Nutbeam 1998, p. 40).

REFERENCES

Allen RE (ed.) (1993) *Oxford Concise Dictionary of Current English*, 8th edn. Oxford: Oxford University Press.

Beresford P (2002) User involvement in research and evaluation: liberation or regulation. *Social Policy and Society* **1**(2): 95–105.

Bradshaw J (1972) The concept of social need. *New Society* **19**: 640–3.

Catford JC (1993) Editorial. *Health Promotion International* **8**: 67–8.

Crafter H (ed.) (1997) Evaluating health promotion activities. In: *Health Promotion in Midwifery Practice Principles and Practice*. London: Arnold, pp. 88–102.

Department of Health (1999) *Patient and Public Involvement in the New NHS*. London: DoH.

Department of Health (2000) *Working Partnerships Consumers in Research. 3rd Annual Report*. London: DoH.

Downie RS, Fyfe C, Tannahill A (1996) *Health Promotion Models and Values*. Oxford: Oxford University Press.

Entwistle VA, Renfrew MJ, Yearley S, Forrester J, Lamont T (1998) Lay perspectives: advantages for health research. *British Medical Journal* **316**: 463–6.

Ewles L, Simnett I (2003) *Promoting Health A Practical Guide*, 5th edn. London: Baillière Tindall.

Hepworth J (1997) Evaluation in health outcomes research: linking theories, methodologies and practice in health promotion. *Health Promotion International* **12**: 233–8.

Katz J, Perberdy A (2001) *Promoting Health Knowledge and Practice*, 2nd edn. London: Palgrave Macmillan.

McQueen DV (2002) The evidence debate: Evaluating evidence for public health interventions. *Journal of Epidemiology and Community Health* **56**: 83–4.

Means R, Smith R (1988) Implementing a pluralistic approach to evaluation in health education. *Policy and Politics* **16**: 17–28.

Naidoo J, Wills J (2000) *Health Promotion Foundations for Practice*, 2nd edn. London: Baillière Tindall.

Nutbeam D (1996) Health outcomes and health promotion: defining success in health promotion. *Health Promotion Journal of Australia* **6**: 58–60.

Nutbeam D (1998) Evaluating health promotion – progress, problems and solutions. *Health Promotion International* **13**: 27–44.

Nutbeam D, Smith C, Catford J (1990) Evaluation in health education, progress, problems and possibilities. *Journal of Epidemiology and Community Health* **44**: 83–9.

Nutbeam D, Smith C, Murphy S, Catford J (1993) Maintaining evaluation designs in long term community based health promotion programs. *Journal of Epidemiology and Community Health* **47**: 123–7.

Potvin L, Gendron S, Bilodea A, Chabot P (2005) Integrating social theory in to public health practice. *American Journal of Public Health* **95**: 591–5.

Rootman I, Goodstadt M, Hyndman B et al. (2001) *Evaluation in Health Promotion Principles and Perspectives*. Copenhagen: WHO.

Sackett DL, Rosenberg WC, Muir Gray JA, Haynes RB, Richardson WS (1996) Evidence based medicine: what it is and what it isn't. *British Medical Journal* **3**: 71–2.

Seedhouse D (2003) *Health Promotion Philosophy, Prejudice and Practice*. Chichester: Wiley.

Tones BK, Tilford S (1994) *Health Education: Effectiveness, efficiency and equity*. London: Chapman & Hall.

Trivedi P, Wykes T (2002) From passive subjects to equal partners. Qualitative review of user involvement in research. *British Journal of Psychiatry* **181**: 468–72.

Valente TW (2002) *Evaluating Health Promotion Programs*. New York: Oxford University Press.

FURTHER READING

International Union for Health Promotion and Education (IUHPE) (1999) *The Evidence of Health Promotion Effectiveness*. A report for the European Commission by the International Union for Health Promotion and Education, Brussels, Luxembourg ECSC-EC-EAEC.

Naidoo J, Wills J (2000) *Health Promotion Foundations for Practice*, 2nd edn. London: Baillière Tindall.

Rootman I, Goodstadt M, Hyndman B et al. (2001) *Evaluation in Health Promotion Principles and Perspectives*. Copenhagen: WHO.

Valente TW (2002) *Evaluating Health Promotion Programs*. New York: Oxford University Press.

6 ATTITUDES, VALUES AND HEALTH BEHAVIOURS

JAN BOWDEN

There are many circumstances in life where, on reflection, it seems unfathomable that an unhealthy lifestyle, e.g. smoking, was not identified sooner. When that unhealthy lifestyle causes a danger to occur such as a pre-term birth the question most commonly asked is 'what could have been done to prevent it happening?' However, prior to the danger becoming a reality, the threat posed by the unhealthy lifestyle is ignored and considered irrelevant. This is an issue with which we have all battled one way or another both as individuals and as midwives. The way in which we act and react when looking at our health depends on many factors such as attitudes and beliefs and their effect on our health behaviour. In examining the factors and understanding how they shape and guide health behaviour, the midwife will be able to deliver more meaningful health promotion. Within this chapter, attitude, values, drives and beliefs are defined and their impact, along with other factors on health behaviour, examined. Using the 'theory of reasoned action' (Ajzen and Fishbein 1980) the relationship between attitudes and health behaviour will be looked at before examining Prochaska and DiClemente's (1984) trans-theoretical approach – one of the most commonly used health behaviour change frameworks.

DEFINING BELIEFS, VALUES, INSTINCTS, DRIVES AND ATTITUDES

Within social psychology it is considered that an individual's behaviour is determined by beliefs, values, instincts, drives and attitudes. All these terms are used within theoretical frameworks of behaviour change and all have considerable importance for the midwife when attempting to facilitate and support a woman changing her health behaviour from unhealthy to healthy. In order for a midwife to undertake these facilitating and supporting roles, the midwife needs to be able to define the terms.

Belief

A belief is a conviction based on information that an individual has about a situation or an item. The individual then attaches attributes to the situation or item. A belief can have positive attributes, for example breastfeeding is best for the baby, or negative attributes that are perceived as positive by the individual, for example smoking will make the baby smaller and the labour will be easier. These beliefs are shaped and influenced by many factors such as personality, family, friends, culture and education, and may not be supported by reliable facts as with the second example mentioned above or by the majority of the population. They are based on the individual's own evaluation of the situation or item and they take time to change (Naidoo and Wills 2000, Katz and Perberdy 2001).

Values

Values are emotional laden convictions, which the individual thinks are important, and cares about passionately. Values are acquired through socialization as a child and as an adult and are influenced by many of the same factors that influence beliefs. Values can alter depending on the environment in which individuals find themselves (Naidoo and Wills 2000, Katz and Perberdy 2001).

Instincts

Sometimes called 'basic instincts', these are present at birth and are required for the individual's survival such as hunger or thirst. They are thought by psychologists to be much more powerful than beliefs and attitudes when motivating behaviour (Katz and Perberdy 2001).

Drives

This term is used to describe the powerful motivating urges triggered by instincts, for example the drive to eat when hungry (Naidoo and Wills 2000).

Attitudes

Within psychology attitudes are considered to be more precise than values or beliefs. The term describes an individual's relatively stable feelings towards a situation or an item. They are formed of three key components.

Cognitive

This is the individual's knowledge and information – it is the belief aspect of attitudes.

Affective

This is concerned with emotions, feelings and preferences.

Behavioural

This is concerned with what the individual can actually do, which is determined to a certain extent by what skills they have and are able to initiate, and under what circumstances.

Attitudes are more difficult to change. A change within any of the three component parts of attitude may initiate a change in behaviour; however, there is no guarantee that this will be the case (McKenna and Davis 2005).

FACTORS AFFECTING BELIEFS, VALUES AND ATTITUDES

As with health and health promotion there are a multitude of factors affecting the development of beliefs, values and attitudes, which relate to our health behaviour both as individuals and as midwives. Family, friends, education, work environment and an individual's social circumstances all play a part in developing our beliefs, values and attitudes towards our health behaviour and the way we go about changing that health behaviour. Research has shown the following areas also to be particularly influential.

Age

Research has shown that generally promoting our health and engaging in positive health behaviours tend to increase the older we get (Cockerham 1997, McDade-Montez et al. 2005). This is particularly relevant when working with young women whose ability to perceive risk is lessened as a result of inexperience and lack of knowledge and skills. Typically this may lead them to engage in negative health behaviours (Social Exclusion Unit (SEU) 1999, Health Development Agency (HDA) 2004).

Gender

Generally women tend to promote their health more than men and to have healthier behaviours, although this depends on the activity (Ewles and Simnett 2003, Verplanken 2005). Men are more likely to exercise and engage in physical activities than women but are more likely to smoke and drink more, although this is beginning to change (McDade-Montez et al. 2005). Having said that, women tend to be wrapped up in promoting the health of their dependants, i.e. children, partners and parents, leaving promotion of their own health at the bottom of the list. When a woman becomes pregnant, the pregnancy may act as a catalyst for change. Concern for the well-being of the unborn child is likely to increase the woman's susceptibility to health messages and adjust her health behaviour consequently. Moreover, it may encourage the woman to sustain that health behaviour after birth (Crafter 1997a, Teenage Pregnancy Unit (TPU) 2003).

Culture

Culture is frequently mentioned as a major influence on the way in which health behaviours are viewed (Ewles and Simnett 2003, McDade-Montez et al. 2005), and yet it is one of the hardest concepts to define in health care. Culture is seen by social anthropologists as the fabric of a society's beliefs, involving religious beliefs, myths, art, manners, dress, etc., which holds that society together and is transmitted through the generations in spoken and unspoken ways. The words 'society' and 'culture' run together. Culture is a part of society, but the same, or a similar, culture can span more than one society. Members of a society tend to live together, or at least have close proximity to each other, whereas members of a culture share ideas and meanings that decide to some extent their beliefs and behaviour, but they may be widely spread geographically. There are dangers in the midwife being unaware of, or misunderstanding, a culture or its manifestation in health behaviour. Perhaps the most serious is that of stereotyping people, when it is assumed that a culture makes all members of the cultural group think, feel and behave in a certain way, e.g. all teenagers are difficult to deal with (Crafter 1997a, Naidoo and Wills 2000).

Peer groups

Our peers are an important factor in helping to shape our beliefs. We share ideas with those around us, and most people feel a need to conform to the social groups to which they feel some attachment, and an important way of 'fitting in' is to share similar thoughts, beliefs and behaviour. Smoking is a good example; outside the home the factor most strongly associated with the uptake of smoking is peer group pressure (Swan et al. 1989, Twigg et al. 2004). The attempts of the midwife to encourage healthier behaviour will to some extent be offset by the social needs of the woman to 'fit' her social group. A change in belief or health behaviour may be hampered by a woman's more overwhelming need to be accepted by her peers (Crafter 1997a). To encourage health behaviour change that may affect an individual's popularity within her social group and perhaps reduce her social support is more likely to persuade the individual simply to ignore the advice. The concept of peer group pressure is especially pertinent for midwives working with women whose friends and social contacts influence their behaviour in major ways, e.g. drugs misusers and teenagers. Although presenting an ethical dilemma to the midwife, the task of challenging peer pressure may be more usefully addressed through a community approach, where change may be slow but where general attitudes, which promote peer pressure and the need to 'fit', can be dealt with more fully (SEU 1999, Cribb and Duncan 2002, TPU 2003).

Personality

The relationship between health behaviour and personality has become increasingly recognized in recent years. Personality is seen as crucial to the way health, childbirth and parenting is interpreted. As with defining health, what 'personality' means also has its problems in that a simple, adequate definition does not exist. Psychologists refer to recurring characteristics and patterns of behaviour in a person that demonstrate their interests, attitudes and abilities, and suggest a relatively constant reaction to the environment (Crafter 1997a). Personality is formed primarily within early family life. It has genetic, social and environmental elements, all of which combine to generate a unique person. Personality theories developed within the field of psychology offer some understanding to the aspects of people's characters. The theories of Sigmund Freud, Abraham Maslow and Carl Rogers are well known and brief resumés of these theories are identified in Box 6.1.

Within health behaviour research the five factor model (FFM) (Costa and McCrae 1992) has been developed to provide a framework by which to understand the influence of personality in health behaviours. The five factors are identified as follows (Costa and McCrae 1992, McDade-Montez et al. 2005).

Neuroticism

This is the predisposition to experience and display negative emotions. Those with high neuroticism are likely to have negative health behaviours.

Extraversion

This is the extent of sociability and interest in others. Those with high extraversion are more likely to have positive health behaviours but strong peer pressure may influence negative health behaviours such as smoking, unsafe sex and drug usage.

Openness

This relates to creativeness, imagination and the readiness to try new experiences. Those reporting high levels of openness may also report negative health behaviours such as drug usage.

Agreeableness

This is the degree of trust in others, to convey positive affect towards them. Those with high agreeableness and conscientiousness were found to have positive health behaviours and a more sustained approach to positive health behaviour changes.

Conscientiousness

This is the degree of dependability, determination and self-control.

The FFM provides a common and organized framework and it highlights the influence of personality traits on an individual's health behaviour. However, the midwife needs to bear in mind that the FFM framework, similar to the theories of personality, gives a limited insight into what makes us the way we are or why we are unpredictable at times (McDade-Montez et al. 2005).

Reflection – 1

Think carefully about a clinical issue where your attitudes, beliefs and values have been challenged, e.g. a 13-year-old booking her first pregnancy, a pregnant smoker in early pre-term labour requesting to leave the ward to have a cigarette, a drug user who leaves her baby on the postnatal ward in search of her next fix. Reflect on your feelings and identify how you dealt with them.

HOW ARE ATTITUDES FORMED?

Attitudes are formed as a reaction to one's own personal characteristics and the social environment; they are determined partly by biological inheritance (McConnell 1980), but are predominantly developed by learning in its broadest sense from birth onwards (Crafter 1997b). Children are primarily exposed to the attitudes of their parents, close relatives and friends, and have a fairly consistent environment in terms of attitudes, values and beliefs. This is because, when couples meet, each is

Box 6.1   The personality theories of Freud, Maslow and Rogers

Sigmund Freud

Freud identifies personality as having three distinct structures:

- id (unconscious inherited processes)
- ego (the guard of the id, requiring behaviour acceptable to the outside world)
- superego (from which the conscience develops).

The individual has defence mechanisms that protect the ego and the superego from conflicts that threaten the status quo of existence. Freud identifies denial, repression and sublimation as examples of the defence mechanisms. He believed that these processes generally went on in the subconscious with only occasional forays into the conscious, and influenced all of our day-to-day thoughts and human interactions. His theories are popular partly because his ideas can be explained simply and followed easily when observing the way people react in different situations.

Abraham Maslow

Maslow developed the widely used 'Hierarchy of needs', which encapsulates the development of personality from birth to adulthood, based on the philosophy that in normal circumstances people are motivated, or moved to achieve more and more sophisticated needs, in order to find self-fulfilment and 'self-actualization' – the feeling of being comfortable with oneself. Maslow's hierarchy is often used to demonstrate the stepping-stones in life's developmental processes.

Midwives will recognize many of the stages mirrored in pregnancy, childbirth and early motherhood, e.g. esteem needs can be met when a woman feels that she has achieved her goals of the birth (be it safe delivery, or perhaps birth with optimal drug usage) or self-fulfilment in reaching her potential. For some women, giving birth and becoming a mother will be their ultimate life experience, described by many as the most important significant event of their life. Maslow's stepping stones offer midwives a framework of care – offering safe care, accepting women and families for what they are as they present themselves to the maternity services, and enhancing women's self-esteem by helping them to explore and understand their experiences.

Carl Rogers

Rogers identified the features of *self-concept* and *positive regard* in his theory of personality. Self-concept depends on how an individual sees him- or herself in the world, how this affects behaviour, and how that individual views the world. Rogers' ideal self-concept is positive regard. Internal anxiety is evoked, he believes, when the individual does not behave or perform in the way expected, and self-esteem is reduced when the self-concept conflicts with behaviour.

(Adapted from Crafter 1997a)

attracted to the other because of shared values and similar socioeconomic and educational backgrounds. Therefore their children, whose early environment is closely controlled by their family and immediate friends, are exposed to a biased sample of life experience. The value of such early experience is in security and continuity at a time when the outside world appears to be a place of contradictions and confusion. It is easy to see how an unsettled family life may affect an individual's early experiences.

Sears (1969) suggested that the critical period for attitude formation, becoming long lasting and harder to alter in a significant or radical way, was between the ages of 12 and 30. The teenage years are a particularly important time for attitude formation, when strong social groups are formed. It is a time of experimentation, excitement and turbulence, and an occasion for shaking off the authority of parents and teachers. It can be divided into two phases: 13–16 years of age when young people push for greater independence from their parents but retain great internal conflicts about dependence and independence, and 16–19 when they wish to forge a separate identity from parents and close family (Chambers et al. 2001). These are key staging points in growing up and entering adulthood. With the move from parental control young people look elsewhere for confirmation of their acceptance within a social group. Usually the one nearest to hand is their own peer group. Normative and behavioural beliefs are aired and re-evaluated; sexuality and the new possibility of reproduction are often areas of great consideration and debate within which attitudes are discussed, shared, formed and changed. Such attitudes and beliefs are not necessarily coherent or constant. It is a time to try out different behaviours, different peer groups and different attitudes. Most will settle, a few years down the line, with attitudes not dissimilar to those of their parents, especially if they had a reasonably happy childhood; however, for those with less happy childhoods the settling phase may take longer or may not occur at all (SEU 1999, Chambers et al. 2001).

Every social group develops norms and expectations to which members are expected to adhere. There is considerable social pressure for individuals to share values, attitudes and behaviours, and to 'fit' in. People tend to mix in many social groups during the same period of their lives, e.g. family, neighbours, workmates, friends from school or a previous job – each may require the adoption of different values to 'fit' in. In order to accommodate these different values, an individual will live with a small amount of discord or feeling out of place, e.g. a teenager may *normatively* agree with friends that sexual freedom is a good thing, while *behaviourally* choosing to remain celibate for the time being without feeling too uncomfortable. However, the need to 'fit' in and conform within a group is very strong, and a divergence in beliefs and values among group members may lead to a break-up and a need to form new friendships where values are re-explored and shared. Where a social group share the same values and attitudes, their relationship is likely to be long lasting, and add much to the psychological well-being of each participating member (Crafter 1997a, 1997b).

On becoming pregnant for the first time, a woman will enter a new social group of 'expectant mothers'. Many women are keen to look for information at this time about their pregnant condition, but along with this information inevitably come other people's values and attitudes. Although the way women accept the new knowledge may be preset by their personality and social environment, major life events often bring with them the propensity for openness to absorb new information and new or reconsidered attitudes, in an attempt to 'fit' in this new social group of mothers. However, the midwife needs to be aware that, for women who are in socially excluded groups, this entry into a new social group may be prevented and cause problems with attitude formation with regard to childbirth and good parenting (Bartley 2005, Janssen and Pfaff 2005).

THE RELATIONSHIP BETWEEN ATTITUDES AND HEALTH BEHAVIOURS

Understanding attitudes has long been felt by many psychologists to be an essential precursor to understanding and attempting to predict people's behaviour, especially in matters of health. It seems obvious that a woman must want to give up smoking, or want to breastfeed, before she actually does it. However, the reverse relationship between attitude and behaviour may be even more complicated (Crafter 1997b, Ewles and Simnett 2003, Proschaska 2005), e.g. a woman may claim to value breastfeeding, and have a positive attitude towards it, but has no intention of breastfeeding her own baby. The complexity of the issue is difficult to disentangle but theories have been developed to explain why individuals behave as they do. These theories include the 'health belief model' (Rosenstock 1966, Becker 1974), the oldest and probably the best known, the 'theory of reasoned action' (Ajzen and Fishbein 1980) and the 'theory of planned behaviour' (Ajzen 1990), which are explained shortly. All these theories may go some way to helping design more realistic health promotion programmes. This is especially so when there is clear-cut evidence identifying the dangers involved in negative health behaviour and there is a patent expectation by the health-care professional that individuals will immediately change their health behaviour because of that evidence. A perfect example of this would be smoking. There is a significant amount of evidence highlighting the negative health effects of smoking, all of which has been well promoted. Yet the smoking figures indicate an increase rather than the expected decrease, especially in young women who are using smoking to control their appetite (Twigg et al. 2004).

In their 'theory of reasoned action' Ajzen and Fishbein (1980) inserted the word 'intention' between attitude and behaviour. They believed that, by discovering a person's intention, rather than their attitude, their behaviour could be more accurately predicted (Ajzen and Fishbein 1980, Ajzen 1988). Crafter (1997b) used this theory in diagrammatic form to show its use within health promotion in midwifery for a woman intending to breastfeed and another intending to use formula feed (Figure 6.1).

Within the 'theory of reasoned action' just two of the multitudes of beliefs held by an individual are identified: behavioural beliefs, i.e. those that make us behave in a certain way; and normative, or desirable, culturally acceptable beliefs. Ajzen and Fishbein (1980) suggest that logical psychological processes link these beliefs by way of our attitude to the behaviour, subjective norm (social pressure) and intention, each stage leading on from the preceding stage. The theory's main conviction is that individuals will weigh up their personal feelings, or attitudes, and the social pressure that they perceive (subjective norm) before arriving at and carrying out their intention to change their health behaviour (or not). Their behaviour is then one of 'reasoned action'.

Ajzen (1990) went on to develop the 'theory of planned behaviour' to incorporate another variable – that of control. In his 'theory of planned behaviour' Ajzen

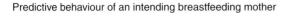

Predictive behaviour of an intending breastfeeding mother

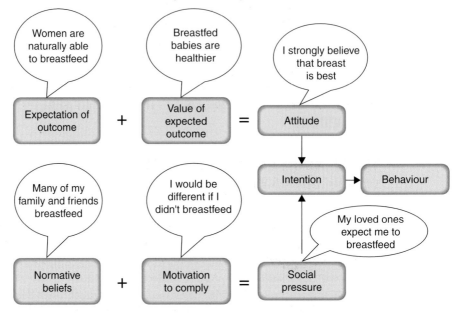

Predictive behaviour of an intending bottle-feeding mother:

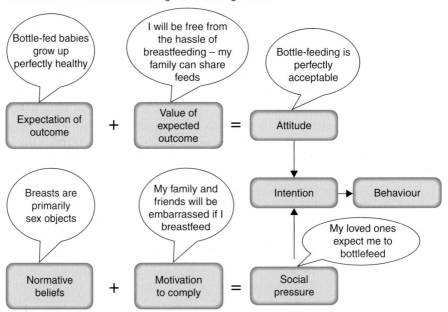

FIGURE 6.1 *Modified theory of reasoned action (modified from Ajzen and Fishbein 1980 by Crafter (1997)). (Reproduced by kind permission.)*

identified that individuals' perceptions of their control over a situation also influenced health behaviours. Individuals differ in the extent to which they think that they can make changes to their lives. Social learning theorists believe that this is a product of an individual's upbringing. Individuals who have been rewarded for their success and have received fair punishment when they have been wrong will have a better belief in their control of their lives than those who have not been rewarded and been unfairly punished (Naidoo and Wills 2000). Although Ajzen and Fishbein (1980) suggest that their theory can be used to predict and understand attitudes and behaviour, the theory does not encompass basic instincts or drives. Nor does it take into account the emotional input, which is often unpredictable. Childbirth is not only a very emotional time for a new mother and her partner, but is also very often an experience where fresh ideas and values are formulated and attitudes changed.

THE TRANSTHEORETICAL APPROACH TO HEALTH BEHAVIOUR CHANGE

Although it is important to acknowledge an individual's attitudes and values in health promotion, and to respect them, it is also essential that a supportive environment be created in which an individual can challenge ideas and question beliefs. The growth of knowledge about ourselves and the outside world aroused by such challenges provides a day-to-day allure in life for the companionship of others, both to confirm our beliefs and, when we feel secure enough, to move on to different levels of knowledge, with which come more complex beliefs and attitudes.

Pregnancy, childbirth and parenting provide a time that requires immense psychological development, when women acquire a great deal of new information, both from the experience of their own pregnancy and from other sources such as family, friends, magazines and health professionals. Although midwives pay great lip service to the importance of giving unbiased information and respecting women's wishes, we also have a moral role in informing women about health-damaging behaviours when and where they may occur. Common examples include information about the dangers to the woman and fetus of continued smoking, alcohol consumption or drug taking in pregnancy, and making sure that women are aware and able to have the opportunity to discuss the advantages to both mother and baby of breastfeeding over formula feeding. The areas of nutrition and exercise in pregnancy are less clear cut in terms of what is healthy, but nevertheless midwives have a duty to encourage discussion of such topics.

To understand how individuals come to change their health behaviours there is a need to differentiate between a change in attitude and a change in behaviour, and to be aware of the time scale involved. In 1984 Prochaska and DiClemente developed a 'trans-theoretical approach'. This approach, developed specifically for smoking cessation, looked for the first time at the actual process undertaken by individuals when changing their health behaviour rather than the factors involved in changing health behaviours and, very controversially for the time, it made clear identification of a relapse stage in light of the evidence showing that long-term smokers took three to four attempts over a 7- to 10-year period before finally quitting (Prochaska and DiClemente 1984). The approach identifies seven stages (Figure 6.2).

1. The pre-contemplation stage

At this point in time the woman has no awareness of a need to change her health behaviour. The midwife, to raise the awareness of the woman, can use health advice

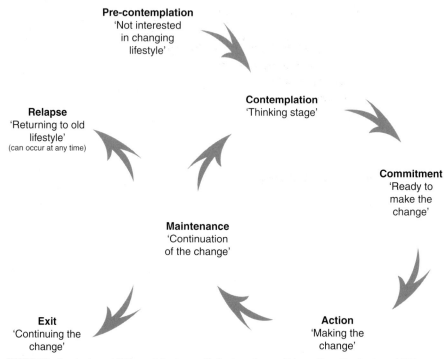

FIGURE 6.2 *Prochaska and DiClemente's stages of behaviour change. (Adapted from Prochaska and DiClemente 1984.)*

and gentle non-judgemental questions about the negative health behaviour. Once she becomes aware the woman then moves to the next stage of the approach. It is important for the midwife to realize that the woman may be hostile to any attempt to discuss the dangers of her negative health behaviour, suggesting that she has yet to reach the pre-contemplation stage (and may indeed never do so). Realistically, it is unlikely that further attempts to discuss cessation will serve a useful purpose, and may even damage the midwife's relationship with the woman. Alternatively she may accept anti-smoking arguments but claim to feel quite powerless to stop. A time span on this is difficult because some women may remain in this stage for many years (Prochaska 2005).

2. The contemplation stage

This is where the health behaviour change starts and may take up to 6 months (Prochaska 2005). The woman, now aware of the side effects of her negative health behaviour, is motivated to think about making the change. She now actively seeks information about the negative health behaviour and the benefits that will come by making a change to it. Empowerment is key to moving through this stage and the midwife can use her considerable skills to facilitate this process, as well as assisting the woman with the collection of information. The midwife must also realize that some of her clients may never move beyond this stage.

3. The commitment stage

A woman entering this stage of the approach is making a serious decision to change her negative health behaviour. The midwife can help the woman by working with her to identify resources and develop action plans, as well as highlighting coping strategies that may help when things get tough. Towards the end of this stage a date on which to commence the change needs to be clearly acknowledged. Prochaska (2005) identifies that this stage usually lasts no more than a month.

4. The action stage

Here the woman is changing the negative health behaviours. She is making explicit modifications to improve her health behaviours and this stage may take up to 6 months (Prochaska 2005). Support during this stage is vital and the midwife can offer support to the woman as well as referral to self-help support groups, and the development of a support group made up of family and friends and identified in the commitment stage of this approach.

5. The maintenance stage

This is when the woman maintains the health behaviour change and prevents a relapse back to her old health behaviour. Here the midwife provides support for the woman by facilitating the woman's use of her action plans and her coping strategies identified in the commitment stage. The woman gains satisfaction from her maintenance of the health behaviour change, which will increase her self-esteem and confidence. Prochaska (2005) highlights that this stage can last for 6 months and beyond.

6. The exit stage

This is where the health behaviour has been successfully changed and maintained by the woman. At this stage the woman is not affected by temptation and has 100 per cent self-efficacy. It is important for the midwife to offer support as required, but it is also important for the midwife to realize that only a small number of women will reach this stage. For most women the best that they will achieve is a lifetime in maintenance stage (Prochaska 2005).

7. The relapse stage

It is important for both the woman and the midwife to realize that this approach will not be successful for everybody at the first attempt. It is also important that relapse is a fact of life when changing health behaviours and it should not be deemed a failure on the part of the woman. Relapse should be evaluated as to its cause and, on starting the approach again, this evaluation can be worked into an action plan and a coping strategy can be developed. This will allow the midwife to offer support, particularly at the point in the approach that the last relapse happened.

SUMMARY OF KEY POINTS

- It is vital to understand how beliefs, values, drives and attitudes affect how individuals form their health behaviour.
- The relationship between attitudes and behaviours is complex. A change within any of the three component parts of attitude may initiate a change in behaviour; however, there is no guarantee that this will be the case.
- Age, gender, culture, peer support and personality are just some of the multitude of factors that influence attitudes and attitude formation.
- Health behaviour theories highlight the factors involved when an individual initiates a change in negative health behaviour.
- Prochaska and DiClemente's trans-theoretical approach identifies the process that an individual goes through during health behaviour change and shows the midwife where their skills can be used.
- Pregnancy is often a time when a woman and her partner are open to new ideas and may change their attitudes as they re-evaluate their lives, learn more about themselves and join a new social group of being parents. The midwife needs to bear in mind that those women in socially excluded groups might find this difficult to achieve.
- Midwives need to be sensitive to the individual's values, the complex issues of health behaviour and the ethical dimensions of attempting to change an individual's values and attitudes.
- Midwives also need to be aware of their own values, beliefs and attitudes, and how that may impact on the care that they give their clients.

REFERENCES

Ajzen I (1988) *Attitudes, Personality and Behaviour.* Milton Keynes: Open University Press.

Ajzen I (1990) The theory of planned behaviour. *Organisational Behaviour and Human Decision Processes* **50**: 179–211.

Ajzen I, Fishbein M (eds) (1980) *Understanding Attitudes and Predicting Social Behaviour.* Englewood Cliffs, NJ: Prentice Hall.

Bartley M (2005) Socio-economic environments. In: Kerr J, Weitkunat R, Moretti M (eds), *ABC of Behavior Change. A guide to successful disease prevention and health promotion.* London: Elsevier Churchill Livingstone, pp. 127–37.

Becker MH (ed.) (1974) *The Health Belief Model and Personal Health Behaviour.* Thorofare, NJ: Slack.

Chambers R, Wakely G, Chambers S (2001) *Tackling Teenage Pregnancy. Sex, culture and needs.* Oxford: Routledge.

Cockerham WC (1997) Lifestyles, social class, demographic characteristics and health behavior. In: Gochman DS (ed.), *Handbook of Health Behavior Research 1: Personal and social determinants.* New York: Plenum Press.

Costa PT Jr, McCrae RR (1992) *Revised NEO Personality Inventory (NEO-PI-R) and NEO Five-Factor Inventory (NEO-FFI) Professional Manual.* Odessa, FL: Psychological Assessment Resources.

Crafter H (1997a) Personal and cultural influences on health. In: Crafter H (ed.), *Health Promotion in Midwifery. Principles and practice.* London: Hodder, pp. 22–33.

Crafter H (1997b) Attitudes, values and behaviour. In: Crafter H (ed.), *Health Promotion in Midwifery. Principles and practice.* London: Hodder, pp. 54–64.

Cribb A, Duncan P (2002) *Health Promotion and Professional Ethics.* London: Blackwell Science.

Ewles L, Simnett I (2003) *Promoting Health: A practical guide*, 5th edn. London: Baillière Tindall.

Health Development Agency (2004) *Teenage Pregnancy: An overview of the research evidence.* London: HDA.

Janssen C, Pfaff H (2005) Psychosocial environments. In: Kerr J, Weitkunat R, Moretti M (eds), *ABC of Behavior Change. A guide to successful disease prevention and health promotion.* London: Elsevier Churchill Livingstone, pp. 153–66.

Katz J, Peberdy A (2001) *Promoting Health: Knowledge and practice*, 2nd edn. London: Macmillan.

McConnell JV (1980) *Understanding Human Behaviour.* New York: Holt, Rinehart & Winston.

McDade-Montez E, Cvengros J, Christensen A (2005) Personality and individual differences In: Kerr J, Weitkunat R, Moretti M (eds), *ABC of Behavior Change. A guide to successful disease prevention and health promotion.* London: Elsevier Churchill Livingstone, pp. 57–70.

McKenna J, Davis M (2005) The problem of behavior change. In: Kerr J, Weitkunat R, Moretti M (eds), *ABC of Behavior Change. A guide to successful disease prevention and health promotion.* London: Elsevier Churchill Livingstone, pp. 29–40.

Naidoo J, Wills J (2000) *Health Promotion. Foundations for practice*, 2nd edn. London: Baillière Tindall.

Prochaska JO (2005) Stages of change, readiness and motivation. In: Kerr J, Weitkunat R, Moretti M (eds), *ABC of Behavior Change. A guide to successful disease prevention and health promotion.* London: Elsevier Churchill Livingstone, pp. 111–23.

Prochaska JO, DiClemente CC (1984) *The Transtheoretical Approach: crossing traditional boundaries of therapy.* Homewood, IL: Dow Jones/Irwin.

Rosenstock I (1966) Why people use health services. *Millbank Memorial Fund Quarterly* **44**: 94–121.

Sears DO (1969) Political behaviour. In: Lindzey G, Aronson E (eds), *Handbook of Social Psychology*, Vol. 5. Reading, MA: Addison-Wesley, pp. 314–458.

Social Exclusion Unit (1999) *Teenage Pregnancy.* London: DoH.

Swan AV, Melia RJ, Fitzsimmons B, Breeze E, Murray M (1989) Why do more boys than girls smoke cigarettes? *Health Education Journal* **48**: 59–64.

Teenage Pregnancy Unit (2003) Sure Start Plus Pilot Programme – National Evaluation of Sure Start Plus. London: Teenage Pregnancy Unit.

Twigg L, Moon G, Walker S (2004) *The Smoking Epidemic in England.* London: HDA.

Verplanken B (2005) Habits and implementation intention In: Kerr J, Weitkunat R, Moretti M (eds), *ABC of Behavior Change. A guide to successful disease prevention and health promotion.* London: Elsevier Churchill Livingstone, pp. 99–110.

FURTHER READING

Kerr J, Weitkunat R, Moretti M (eds) (2005) *ABC of Behavior Change. A guide to successful disease prevention and health promotion.* London: Elsevier Churchill Livingstone.

Rollnick S, Mason P, Butler C (1999) *Health Behaviour Change – A guide for practitioners.* London: Churchill Livingstone.

INFORMATION GIVING IN HEALTH PROMOTION

VICKY MANNING

Health promotion was virtually unknown before the 1970s and now health information is everywhere, on television and radio, in shops, in newspapers and presented on high street billboards. Much of what we consume, wash in, wear or drive has a health or lifestyle message selling it. Health messages can range from the fruit and vegetables five-a-day campaign to facecreams that remove the signs of ageing and keep you feeling young. Health information is provided in a myriad of different formats (often within the health belief model), and can be influenced by many different elements such as who is sponsoring the campaign, the time available to present the information and the groups being targeted. The ability to provide and assess the quality of information is an important skill for anyone undertaking health promotion activities. The aim of this chapter is to explore the different formats used to provide information in health promotion and how the quality of information given or received can be assessed.

COMMUNICATING HEALTH

The terms 'health promotion' and 'health education' have been used interchangeably. Today it is a generally considered that health promotion is the broad umbrella that tries to facilitate access to a healthy life for everyone. It encompasses transport, housing, environment and agriculture, to name but a few. Health education is predominately considered to be providing information to an individual or group to facilitate them to make informed choices about their lifestyles.

Communication contributes to all aspects of disease prevention, health promotion and health education for individuals, communities and whole populations. Health communication many occur in different areas such as schools, home and work, and in many different formats such as the mass media, flyers, newsletters, advertising and posters. The choice of format for the presentation of information depends on many points such as what the topic is, whom the target group is, who is planning to give the information, where the information is being given and the amount of time planned/available.

It is known that using more than one form of communication is more effective in increasing understanding, than using only one (Kerr et al. 2005), e.g. if providing information on breastfeeding to a group of women, a midwife may discuss the topic with the women, provide leaflets, show a video, provide some website addresses and invite a woman who is breastfeeding to come to talk about her experiences.

No matter how good the communication a point to remember is that, even though information is provided, people may not be ready to hear it. There are elements that can affect how messages are received and interpreted such as it may not be a good time in their lives or they may not want to be told how to live their lives or for others to make decisions for them (Department of Health (DoH) 2004). Part of the ability to interpret health messages is the concept of risk and the instant gratification that some lifestyles (often unhealthy) produce. The health belief model assumes that people will alter their behaviour as shown in the following example:

- At risk of contracting a disease: a woman will take action to prevent cancer, e.g. have a cervical smear. Communicating the availability of the screening programme is vital for this to happen.
- Experiencing symptoms, such as postcoital bleeding may be a cue for someone who may not have felt 'at risk' before to take action, i.e. have a cervical smear. Publicity of what the symptoms are and where to go if concerned is part of the strategy for this screening programme.
- The risk is understood, so she goes and has a cervical smear. Cues may have been taken from mass media campaigns or something that she read in a magazine, the realization that she may be at risk, prompting action.

Not picking up these cues can affect how messages are sought, received and interpreted. Midwives need to be proactive in their health education. It is no good waiting for women to ask for advice; you need to ask questions and seek information from the women and their families. Finding out the woman's and the family's opinions on health-related topics may help you to find out about the family and their social circumstances. This may give some guidance or clues to how information that is given may be interpreted, and any barriers that may affect the woman's or her family's ability to take action, such as the costs, transport links or the time-consuming nature of going to the health centre (Kerr et al. 2005). It will usually take more than one session for people to change behaviour and the information needs to be backed up with materials to take home and review at leisure. This information may not be used immediately but may play a part in behaviour change in the future.

ENSURING QUALITY OF INFORMATION

Midwives give information on a variety of topics, to many different women throughout their working day. There is so much to say and so little time that it can be difficult to know where to begin. When giving information, there are two elements to pay attention to: the quality of the presentation and the quality of the information given. Midwives need to be aware that, however information is provided, there is an element of persuasion or 'manipulation' from the person providing it. This occurs in three main ways:

1. The amount of information given, which is influenced by the quantity of the information and the time allotted to provide it. Choices need to be made by the person providing the

information as to which bits to leave in and which bits to take out. This needs to be considered carefully and information not provided mindlessly in a habitual manner.

2. Framing the message, what words are used and where the emphasis is given, e.g. if you lose weight you are less likely to develop diabetes, or you are still at risk of diabetes even if you lose weight. Both are correct, but one sounds more upbeat than the other. How the health risk or health change is presented can 'manipulate' how the person receiving the information perceives it and this, in turn, may influence decision-making and health behaviours. Decide in advance what is to be related to the woman or family and construct the message accordingly.

3. The order in which the information is given can also influence perceptions. People tend to remember information at the beginning of the conversation, and forget the last bits; this is particularly true if it is bad news. If the topic is considered unimportant, however, the end of the message will be remembered more than the beginning. (Witte 1994).

The quality of presentation has been discussed; now the quality of the information itself needs to be reviewed. This is a big issue because there is a consistent bombardment of 'health' messages all day – information is provided by many different parties, e.g. governments wanting to provide health messages or information on screening interventions, drug companies wanting to sell products, and this may mean that the quality of the information varies. Quality assurance is a concept familiar to most and it is of particular importance when discussing information provision. Quality is relevant for any mode of communication used, be it verbal, film, video or radio.

In 2000 the Department of Health published the Bristol report that looked at medical standards. It recommended the following:

- Information on treatment should be given in a variety of forms and in stages and reinforced over time (recommendation 4).
- Information should be tailored to individual needs, circumstances and wishes (recommendation 5).
- Information is to be based on current available evidence with a summary, which is comprehensible to the client (recommendation 6).
- Modes of providing information, whether leaflets, video, tapes or CDs, should be regularly updated and developed with the help of patients (recommendation 6).
- Clients should receive guidance on sources of information available on the internet that are reliable and of good quality (recommendation 9).

Although not specifically developed for health promotion, these concepts are fundamental to public health and health promotion.

Exercise – 1

Think about your communication with women and their families. Reflect on how you feel your communication measures up to the requirements suggested above.

Before the Bristol report, the Centre for Health Information Quality (CHIQ) was established in 1997. Its major role was in accrediting health information produced by the NHS and other agencies that provide health information, such as Macmillan

Cancer Relief and Discovery Health, for public use (Hain 2004). The three key elements they identify for quality are accuracy, clarity and relevance.

Accuracy

- Consistency: not contradicting itself, consistent layout and brand identifiable, e.g. logos.
- Continuity: information presented in the context of other resources, e.g. is it part of a series, are other resources clearly signposted?
- Current: is the information up to date? Is the date clearly presented, are references or sources of information dated?
- Reliability: is the information evidence based?

Clarity

- Appearance of text: one font used throughout, no over-use of bold font.
- Presentation: information summarized, bullet pointed, good line spacing, clearly labelled diagrams and images, style maintained throughout.
- Content: sentences of not more than 20 words, jargon avoided, specialist terms or abbreviations explained.

Relevance

- Accessible: does the information meet the needs of the patient? Is it available in other languages and formats and is this information provided?
- Appropriate: does it meet the needs of the target group?
- Patient involvement: has the information been designed with input from patients and the public?

There is a toolkit available at www.nhsidentity.nhs.uk/patientinformationtoolkit.

Exercise – 2

- Acquire some leaflets on a health topic that interests you and that the women in your area may access.
- Using the quality attributes compare them for accuracy, clarity and relevance.
- How easy was this to do?
- How much time did it take to achieve a good review of the leaflets you chose?
- Do you think that you could do this regularly to ensure that your clients are receiving high-quality information?

Similar tools to assess the quality of health information have been created by others. Eng and Gustafson (1999) suggest that information is high quality if seen to be accurate, current, valid, appropriate, intelligible and free of bias. The last aspect is particularly important where sponsors are used to pay for the leaflets, airtime, billboard space, etc. The Office of Disease Prevention and Health Promotion (2000) has detailed the attributes that they feel are necessary for effective health communication:

- Accuracy: valid content without errors of fact, interpretation or judgement.
- Availability: delivered or placed where the audience can access it.

- Balance: where appropriate, the content presents the benefits and risks, and recognizes different and valid perspectives on the issue.
- Consistency: internally consistent and consistent with other information sources.
- Cultural competence: design, implementation and evaluation that account for special issues for select groups.
- Evidence based: relevant reviewed scientific evidence.
- Reach: content gets to or is available to the largest possible number of people in the target group.
- Reliability: source of the content is credible and the content is kept up to date.
- Repetition: the delivery and access to content are continued or repeated, to reinforce the impact and to reach new generations.
- Timeliness: content is provided or available when the audience is most receptive or in need of specific information.
- Understandability: the reading or language level and format are appropriate for the specific audience.

All of these quality tools require time and effort to use and are intended for the professional appraiser. When women read leaflets they may need to discuss them, which can take time. You may need to be put aside time to review the quality of information provided by your department so that you can discuss the issues with the woman with confidence. Face-to-face discussion is not especially easy to achieve and requires a variety of skills. Below are some suggestions for midwives using and reviewing different modes of communication.

FACE-TO-FACE COMMUNICATION

Pregnant women and new parents learn about birth and parenthood in different ways. One main source will be midwives who are in an ideal position to provide health information (Royal College of Midwives 2001). Midwives spend a great deal of their time in face-to-face communication with women, couples and families. Midwives require effective communication because good communication can make a person feel valued and listened to and improve understanding. Effective communication underpins health information, it reduces anxiety and improves understanding which, in turn, helps clients to make choices (National Cancer Institute 1989).

For verbal communication four key elements are vital for quality:

1. To listen carefully: midwives are faced with a challenge in that the Government is setting targets to be met, which in a way dictates the information to be provided to women. This should not, however, stop midwives finding out what information individual women want. Communication is not all one way and should involve finding out what the needs of the client or the community are (Unwin et al. 1997). Some clients may require help from the midwife to articulate their needs, because this may be a new concept for them. Midwives need to be prepared to 'listen' to women. Listening is a skill often under-estimated and is more than the ability to hear. It is interpreting the verbal and non-verbal communication that is taking place. The listener is required to give the person speaking time to express their opinion and needs. For some, voicing their own needs is not easy and the listener can help by paying attention, being encouraging, paraphrasing what is being said, reflecting feelings and meanings, and then summing up to ensure that what has been said has been understood (Ewles and Simnett 2003).

2. Explain things clearly, think carefully about what message is to be given and give it in an easily understood manner. It may require the use of written material or video, etc. to reinforce the information.
3. Show respect for what the client or family has to say. Communication is rarely effective without respect being overtly shown. This incorporates acceptance of the woman and her family without judgement of who they are or their lifestyle.
4. Spend enough time with the client.
   (Office of Disease Prevention and Health Promotion 2000)

Crafter (1997) has given a few suggestions on how to facilitate communication in midwifery further.

Genuineness

The woman knows that she is dealing with a 'real' person, so games and ploys are not necessary and then personally meaningful communication can take place.

Empathy

Empathy means taking seriously the ideas, beliefs and concerns of the other party. It is the ability to put oneself in another person's position and see things from their perspective.

Kindness

Small acts of kindness are often remembered for a long time, as are perceived acts of unkindness.

Honesty

Most people value honesty because it engenders trust. Dishonesty or concealment of information is usually discovered fairly quickly, and this can have long-term serious consequences for the woman in her dealings with all health professionals who have future contact with her.

Diplomacy

Diplomacy is necessary for skilled communication, especially when there is bad news to impart. It is a skill that develops with experience, often of previously poorly managed situations, and practice.

Reflection

Reflect on personal biases and prejudices that may affect the way you communicate with some women and their families. Also reflection on practice can transform knowledge and experience into personal learning – education and professional care become more of a partnership between midwife and mother.

Balancing skills

Part of effective communication is being able to balance when to listen and when to provide information. Sometimes women will desire information, or they may need support for a decision that they have made about their care.

Standing back

Standing back from a situation is a skill developed through self-awareness and experience. It allows the woman to make her choice and live with it, and respects her for her right to choose. For the midwife it means not being personally affronted if a woman chooses to continue to smoke, or partake in health-damaging behaviour, but continuing to provide support that is non-judgemental of the person.

Non-English speaking

People with limited command of English often find it difficult to gain adequate information about health and may not be aware of how to access health care (Phul et al. 2003). For this population it has been found that the one-to-one meeting is useful, although translators can make the information stilted. The use of verbal presentations, video and leaflets in the relevant language has all been found to be very useful to improve communication.

INFORMATION FROM THE MEDIA

Each format for providing information has influence and the most influential is the mass media. Getting health messages across via the media has grown enormously in the last 30 years. The public now receive a vast amount of health messages through this mode, through watching television, listening to the radio and reading magazines, newspapers and leaflets, and seeing billboards and posters.

Messages about health are also provided as entertainment on the television and are considered to be a powerful tool for reaching a wide audience. Many soap operas have health messages within them such as Alma dying of cervical cancer in *Coronation Street*, or Mark diagnosed with HIV in *EastEnders*. Unfortunately 'bad' behaviours are not usually condemned and solutions are not necessarily offered in these programmes. If television shows convey inaccurate information or risky behaviour, but do not show the possible consequences of that behaviour, viewers may suffer negative effects (Beck et al. 2003). The mass media can provide information to a wide population quickly, giving reminders of the effects of health-damaging behaviours and the benefits of adopting healthy behaviours (Naidoo and Wills 2000). In the USA, a survey of 2636 people over the age of 18 in 1999 reported that a high proportion of daytime television viewers gained health information from soap operas. It also reported that health information was received from many different media formats: 83 per cent of the respondents reported information gained from television, 78 per cent from newspapers or magazines, 71 per cent from direct communication with other people, 24 per cent from the radio and 13 per cent from the internet (Center for Disease Control and Prevention 1999).

Raising awareness on its own is unlikely to lead to long-term changes in the health behaviour of individuals (Ewles and Simnett 2003). The value of the acquisition of such knowledge is therefore debatable. However, as health becomes more prominent in the media and with television programmes such as the BBC's *Fat Nation*, it could be argued that the subsequent widespread public awareness makes people discuss health more. This may motivate people and result in some change in their lifestyles (DoH 2004). What is demonstrated by the US survey, and recognized by the British Government, is the enormous potential that the media have to convey messages to large audiences and the responsibility programme makers have to ensure that story lines and any information given are as accurate as possible.

The use of mass media to convey health messages has had mixed success (Tones and Tilford 2001, Slater 2005). Many of you may still remember the HIV 'don't die of ignorance' campaign in the early 1980s. This particular campaign was run on the television, radio and posters, and leaflets were delivered to every home. It was very successful at the time, but the message is now fading into the past, demonstrating the short-term effects of messages if they are not constantly followed up and reinforced. The Government, at present, is running the '5-A-DAY' campaign. This uses many different modes of communication to convey this health message to a wide spectrum of the public. The awareness of the campaign in 2002 was 52 per cent; in 2003, this had risen to 59 per cent, with the consumption of fresh fruit rising by 5.8 per cent (DoH 2004).

Exercise – 3

- What do you think of the above figures for awareness of the '5-A-DAY' campaign?
- How aware were you of this campaign?
- Do you think that the women and their families whom you meet daily are aware?
- How can you increase their awareness of the campaign and the value of eating five portions of fruit or vegetables a day?

With health as entertainment (there is at least one health education programme or documentary on a health-related issue every day), it is often the bad news that makes good press. Messages that generate some increased awareness of health issues are often the 'bad news' with shocking headlines. This can provide a distorted message to the public of the issue being discussed (Ewels and Simmett 2003). In addition, viewers may misinterpret or misunderstand the message being provided, whether positive or negative, which can be quite difficult to counteract, because viewers may think that the information is correct, especially if provided by an 'expert'. Midwives need to take time to listen to the perceived message and then to provide an alternative view, which may need to be backed up with written material.

Leaflets and the printed word

Clients have been shown to remember only about 20 per cent of what they are told during a medical consultation. Up to 50 per cent of what is spoken about will be retained if written information is also provided (Moult and Frank 2004). There should be no complacency that the information has been provided just because a leaflet has been given out. In 2003, 5.2 million adults in England lacked basic literacy skills. In a survey of the readability of patient information in palliative care it was found that 64 per cent of leaflets were understood by 40 per cent of the population. Sixty per cent found it difficult to understand the leaflets (DoH 2004). This means that some women may not be able to read a leaflet and many women may be able to read the leaflet but find it too difficult to understand.

Leaflets are considered expert opinion but there is some evidence to show that different leaflets on the same topic are not always consistent in the information they provide, e.g. use different terminology, different risk factors, etc., and may cause confusion and distress (Jones 2003). This is a potential problem with the quality as already identified above. There is constant tension about what information should be provided – general advice or specific information – and how much (Payne 2002). The answer to these questions depends on the target audience and the aim of the leaflet. When giving out a leaflet, the midwife should be aware of its content and so be able to talk to the woman or her family about the contents and places where they may go for further information.

Exercise – 4

- Look again at the leaflets you reviewed for quality.
- What information do they present: general or specific?
- How useful is the information to the target audience?
- Do the leaflets have suggestions or contact numbers for further information?
- If so, follow these up and see if these links are working, valid and useful.

The manufacturers of health products advertise their goods in many different formats and health information leaflets are one form. Their vested interest in selling their products can potentially make the information provided biased. The way in which it is presented as fact may confuse the customers so that they assume that the information is wholly correct. Even if the information is correct, there may be bias within the text towards their product. This can include 'health promotion' leaflets that may be available to women in chemists, doctor's surgeries, health centres and antenatal clinics.

Leaflets are widely available and are a useful way of providing information to women and their families, or to back up information that they have received. However, they are not a substitute for discussing issues with women and families, although they can be used effectively to introduce topics before discussion, such as HIV screening during the antenatal period, or as a memory aid for subjects such as postnatal exercises. Health professionals have a responsibility to ensure that good quality leaflets are provided and that those of poorer quality are not given out.

INFORMATION TECHNOLOGY

Information technology (IT) is the mechanical and electronic means of communication. Increasing confidence is being placed in its potential power to transform communication with clients. IT has grown so much in recent years not only because of the great leap forward in the development of technology, but also because there is a great hunger for information and a need to store and retrieve it efficiently. Books, videos, television and newspapers provide excellent everyday modes of mass communication, but computers, CDs and DVDs, the internet and telecommunications such as mobile phones allow communication to be ever more efficient. The convergence of all the different media formats has created a communication highway, with an increasing amount of health information and support services available at the press of a button (Crafter 1997).

The internet is one form of interactive mass media that has advanced rapidly in a very short space of time. Searching for health information using a search engine is the third most common use of the internet (Bernstam et al. 2005). The internet may have advantages such as access to information that is specific and personal, access to information on demand, information being distributed widely and updated easily. It also provides more choice, access to support from health-care providers and communication with others with similar problems to exchange and share information (Office of Disease Prevention and Health Promotion 2000).

The World Wide Web has the potential to alter health information provision. There is a vast amount of health-related information available to just about everybody, and this is only the start, but this information needs to be assessed for quality. There is the potential that information might be misleading, inaccurate or inappropriate and consumers accessing the information may make choices based on that information, with no professional guidance. Care needs to be taken when comments such as 'I want to share my experience', 'this site is sponsored by' and 'this is a summary of other information' are seen (Roberts and Copeland 2001). There are a great many tools available for consumers to use to assess the quality of the information being provided, but they have many different parts to them and require good reading and comprehension skills. In one review of 273 instruments none was found to be user friendly (Bernstam et al. 2005). Midwives will need to be aware of this when meeting women who have health information from the internet, and must be able to support clients accessing the information so that they can use it appropriately and safely (Rogers and Mead 2004, Bernstam et al. 2005).

Exercise – 5

- Use a search engine of your choice to type in a health topic in which you are interested, e.g. diabetes, congenital heart defect.
- How many 'hits' did you get?
- Access the first five and read the information provided:
  - do any of them have a quality assurance logo?
  - if they do have a logo try to find the quality assurance tool used and critique it
  - if they do not have a logo, do your own assessment for quality using the CHIQ format
  - in your opinion how useful is the information that you found for a layperson?

Another issue that needs to be considered is access to the technology. The internet may be free in the library, but it is not free at home. Not everyone can or wants to own a computer and internet connection. We may be moving towards yet another area of inequality, identified in the USA as the digital divide (Office of Disease Prevention and Health Promotion 2000). There are reasons to suspect that low-education, low-income groups are the least likely to access information and some may have difficulty using the technology. There is also, as with the leaflets, the requirement to have reading and comprehension skills to make sense of the information provided, and a requirement to have the technical skills to acquire the information. In one survey it was found that 53 per cent of adults did not have the required skills to use IT (DoH 2004).

For midwives the internet may be an invaluable resource, but ensure the quality of the information. If web pages are being recommended, make sure that they are checked because they change frequently. Suggesting use of the internet for acquiring information comes with a responsibility to remind the users that the information provided in chat rooms and on some sites may be of a poor quality or inaccurate. Midwives who suggest use of the internet should make themselves available to discuss issues that may be raised from the information found and to review the quality of the information retrieved.

SUMMARY OF KEY POINTS

- When giving health information, think about using more than one format; it may help to make the message more understandable, e.g. verbal, written, use of video- or audio-tapes.
- Before providing information to women or their families, consider carefully what you want to convey, where the information is being given and the amount of time that you have.
- Midwives need to listen to women to find out their personal attitudes and opinions on health. Information may need to be repeated several times because, depending on the circumstances of the woman, she may or may not be ready to accept or use the information at that point.
- The quality of the information is an important factor. Quality assurance is a time-consuming practice, but worth doing to ensure that clients have the best available information on which to base any health choices.
- Quality applies to all modes of information provision. It is particularly relevant in mass media and the internet.
- The mass media are a very powerful tool for providing information to a wide audience, but misinterpretations or misunderstandings can, and do, arise.
- The internet provides access to vast amounts of information, some of which may be of poor quality. Midwives need to evaluate the quality of information that they may be given by women.
- Spending time with women who bring information with them from the internet or who want to discuss something that they saw on television can be time-consuming, but will help women to make more informed choices.

REFERENCES

Beck V, Huang GC, Pollard WE, Johnson TJ (2003) TV drama viewers and health information. Paper presented at American Public Health Association 131st annual meeting and exposition, San Francisco, CA: www.cdc.gov/communication/surveys/surv2001.pdf (accessed February 2005).

Bernstam EV, Shelton DM, Walji M, Meric-Berstam F (2005) Instruments to assess the quality of health information on the World Wide Web: what can our patients actually use? *International Journal of Medical Informatics* **74**: 13–19.

Center for Disease Control and Prevention (1999) Porter Novelli health styles survey: www.cdc.gov/communication/surveys/surv1999.htm (accessed February 2005).

Crafter H (ed.) (1997) Midwives and communication. In: *Health Promotion in Midwifery: Principles and practice*. London: Arnold.

Department of Heath (2000) *Final Report of the Bristol Royal Infirmary Inquiry*: www.bristol-inquiry.org.uk/final_report/index.htm (accessed January 2005).

Department of Health (2004) *Choosing Health*. London: DoH.

Eng TR, Gustafson DH (eds) (1999) *Wired for Health and Wellbeing: The emergence of interactive health communication*. Washington DC: US Department of Health and Human Services. Cited in Office of Disease Prevention and Health Promotion (2000).

Ewles L, Simnett I (2003) *Promoting Health: A practical guide*. London: Baillière Tindall.

Hain T (2004) Health information appraised for quality. *Health Expectations* **7**: 85.

Jones SA (2003) A review of the consistency of breast cancer screening pamphlets produced by health authorities in Australia. *Health Education* **103**: 166–76.

Kerr J, Weitkunat R, Moretti M (2005) *ABC of Health Behavior: A guide to successful disease prevention and health promotion*. Edinburgh: Elsevier.

Moult B, Frank L (2004) Ensuring quality information for patients: development and preliminary validation of a new instrument to improve the quality of written health care information. *Health Expectations* **7**: 165–75.

Naidoo J, Wills J (2000) *Health Promotion Foundations for Practice*, 2nd edn. Edinburgh: Baillière Tindall.

National Cancer Institute (1989) *Making Health Communications Work*. Washington, DC: US Department of Health and Human Services. Cited in Office of Disease Prevention and Health Promotion (2000).

Office of Disease Prevention and Health Promotion (2000) Healthy people 2010 Health Communication, Chapter 11. US Department of Health and Social Services 11-3 to 11-22: www.healthypeople.gov/document/pdf/volume1/11Healthcom.pdf (accessed October 2005).

Payne SA (2002) Balancing information needs: dilemmas in producing patient leaflets. *Health Informatics Journal* **8**: 174–9.

Phul A, Bath PA, Jackson MG (2003) The provision of information by health promotion units to people of Asian origin living in the UK. *Health Informatics Journal* **9**: 39–56.

Roberts JM, Copeland KL (2001) Clinical websites are currently dangerous to health. *International Journal of Medical Informatics* **62**: 181–7.

Rogers A, Mead N (2004) More than technology and access: primary care patients' views on the use and non-use of health information in the Internet age. *Health and Social Care in the Community* **12**: 102–10.

Royal College of Midwives (2001) *The Midwife's Role in Public Health. Position Paper 24*. London: RCM.

Slater M (2005) Mediated communication. In: Kerr J, Weitkunat R, Moretti M (eds), *ABC of Health Behavior: A guide to successful disease prevention and health promotion*. Edinburgh: Elsevier, pp. 303–14.

Tones K, Tilford S (2001) *Health Education: Effectiveness, efficiency and equity*, 3rd edn. Cheltenham: Nelson Thornes.

Unwin N, Carr S, Leeson J (1997) *An Introductory Study Guide to Public Health and Epidemiology*. Buckingham: Open University Press.

Witte K (1994) The manipulative nature of health communication research: ethical issues and guideline. *American Behavioral Scientist* **38**: 385–93.

FURTHER READING

Antony D (1996) *Health on the Internet.* Oxford: Blackwell.
Watterson A (2003) *Public Health in Practice.* Basingstoke: Palgrave Macmillan.

INTERNET SITES

Discovery Health: www.discoveryhealth.co.uk – Provides a range of health information services.
Patient.co.uk: www.patient.co.uk – Provides leaflets on health-related topics.

8 HEALTH PROMOTION IN MIDWIFERY TRAINING

VICKY MANNING

In Chapter 1 the intrinsic role of the midwife within health promotion has been recognized and discussed in some detail. When formulating a new curriculum for a 'direct entry' programme of Diploma in Midwifery Studies in the Florence Nightingale School of Nursing and Midwifery, King's College London, the health promotion aspect was considered very carefully. The overall aim of the curriculum is to 'define standards that will enable childbearing women and babies to achieve optimum health and wellbeing' (Department of Health (DoH) 2003a) and there is much that has influenced the creation of this curriculum. To achieve this aim, the professional and Government agendas need to be followed and the student as an individual needs to be acknowledged.

This chapter looks at the preparation of students for their health promotion role within one programme of midwifery education.

PHILOSOPHY OF CARE AND EDUCATION IN THE CURRICULUM

Pregnancy is not an illness and midwives provide care and support for a generally healthy population who are undergoing a normal but transforming life event. Central to the philosophy of the programme leading to the Diploma in Midwifery Studies and registration as a midwife is the acknowledgement that each woman and her experiences are unique. For each woman care delivery should be equitable, accessible, acceptable and individual, and these are all the elements of woman-centred care called for in the key texts by the House of Commons Health Committee (HOC 1992) and that called *Changing Childbirth* (DoH 1993). For midwives to be able to provide flexible woman-centred care, they need to be knowledgeable, self-aware, non-judgemental, reflective and adaptable. The varied aspects that influence health, such as socioeconomic, cultural, physical and psychological factors, need to be acknowledged, along with the woman's individual needs and wishes.

Care should be evidence based and planned in partnership with the woman and where necessary other health professionals. This requires communication, negotiation and collaborative skills. The team of midwifery tutors believe that appropriate care given in a supportive manner enhances a woman's self-confidence and helps to achieve the optimal outcome for the woman, her baby and her family. The education process aims to embrace this philosophy and produce competent, skilful practitioners who have developed analytical and critical abilities, which can then be translated into high-quality holistic care.

Learning is a dynamic, interactive process of the student, lecturer and clinician. It is also a process that is the responsibility of the individual. A holistic approach helps the students to grow in self-awareness and responsibility, so developing their potential as adult learners. This, in turn, will facilitate them in acknowledgement of the concept that learning is a life-long process, so they will continue to develop as individuals and midwives post-registration.

WHAT INFORMED THE CURRICULUM?

There are two reports that recommended fundamental changes to the way midwives work: the report of the HOC (1992) and *Changing Childbirth* (DoH 1993). These two documents called for a maternity service that was flexible and provided woman-centred care to meet the needs of the individual woman and her family.

From these papers have come more documents and policies that guide and inform maternity services. It has been shown that women value community-based maternity services higher than hospital-based services (Audit Commission 1997, 1998). The drive has been towards a more holistic approach to care, which means that midwives need to provide flexible care both in the hospital setting and increasingly in the community. This, by its very nature, has put midwives more in the frontline for health promotion activities.

Further recommendations on the provision of maternity services are outlined in *The New NHS: Modern and dependable* (DoH 1997), *A First Class service: Quality in the new NHS* (DoH 1998) and *Towards Safer Childbirth* (Royal College of Obstetrics and Gynaecology/Royal College of Midwives (RCM) 1999). Recommendations include midwives providing more care in the community, ensuring that services make a difference to women in their local communities and addressing inequalities as much as possible. This concept of midwives influencing local communities was built on in the document *Making a Difference: Strengthening the nursing and midwifery contribution to health and healthcare* (DoH 1999). In this document, it is suggested that there are increasing opportunities for midwives to initiate health promotion strategies, which address health inequalities for childbearing women and their families.

As a result of the documents above and *The NHS Plan* (DoH 2000), 10 taskforces were created to plan the reality of the NHS plan. One of these was the Children's Taskforce; one of its responsibilities was to create the *National Service Framework for Children, Young People and Maternity Services* (called the NSF throughout this chapter). This very influential document was not published when the curriculum was developed but, since publication, it has influenced the day-to-day running of the curriculum. However, the preliminary findings had been published and these were used as part of the curriculum planning. The overall aim of the NSF is to:

- improve services
- tackle inequalities
- enhance partnership.

Major themes include health promotion and prevention of illness, early identification, and effective management of problems, empowerment, self-management and family support, and child-/woman-centred care (DoH 2003a).

The following were the main points that emerged from the findings:

1. The promotion of best outcome for women, babies and families requires maternity services that are women focused, involving users in all aspects of service provision.
2. The promotion of normality, balanced with early identification and management of relevant social, medical and psychiatric problems.
3. Services need to meet nationally agreed standards of care; this requires enhancing communication and teamwork between health-care professionals and social workers, and women.
4. Women need individualized care plans based on informed choice and agreed by the women and health-care professionals. These should reflect the needs and preferences of the woman and her family, should offer appropriate, accessible and realistic options for place of birth, appropriate care and support in labour, and are backed up by coordinated emergency care provision for both the mother and the baby.
5. Postnatal care should be structured to give the newborn the best possible start and help the mother to recover fully from the birth, both physically and mentally.
6. Support and information given in the antenatal period should be built on, and new tailor-made plans created if necessary.
7. All women need to have appropriate access to community, hospital and/or specialist services.

Linked to the NSF is the document *Improvement, Expansion and Reform: The next three years, priorities and planning framework 2003–2006* (DoH 2003b). This has quite specific preliminary targets:

- A 1 per cent reduction per year in the proportion of women continuing to smoke in pregnancy, focusing especially on women from disadvantaged groups as a move towards the national target of reducing, by at least 10 per cent, the gap in infant mortality between social classes IV and V and the rest of the population by 2010.
- Deliver an increase of 2 per cent per year in breastfeeding initiation rate, focusing especially on women from disadvantaged groups.
- Achieve agreed local reduction targets in teenage conception.
- Improve access to services for disadvantaged groups and areas, particularly sexual health services and antenatal services.

Recommendations from the *Fitness to Practice Report* (United Kingdom Central Council for Nursing, Midwifery and Health Visiting (UKCC) 1999) and *Organisation with a Memory* (DoH 2001) highlight the challenges faced by the midwifery profession when providing a quality service that promotes partnership with women and other care professionals. This, in turn, has raised concern about defining the specific competencies expected at the point of midwifery registration. In 2000 the UKCC published *Guidelines for Pre-registration Midwifery Programmes* (adopted by the Nursing and Midwifery Council (NMC) 2004). This provides generic midwifery competencies, which have been used to form a basis for the clinical assessment tool and to inform the content of modules, providing a theory/practice link (see Box 8.1 for education standards).

> **Box 8.1 Standards of education to achieve the NMC standards of proficiency**
>
> These are the guiding principles that establish the philosophy and values underpinning the Nursing and Midwifery Council's (NMC's) requirements to entry to the midwives' part of the register and should be reflected in midwifery programmes. The education of student midwives will:
>
> - demonstrate a woman-centred approach to care, based on partnership, which respects the individuality of the woman and her family
> - promote ethical and non-discriminatory practices
> - reflect the quality dimension of care through the setting and maintenance of appropriate standards
> - take into account the changing nature and context of midwifery practice
> - base practice on the best available practice

The courses in the programme reflect the health promotion role of the midwife, as outlined in the many documents mentioned above, and endeavours to prepare students for their role as autonomous practitioners. Documents that have been published since the curriculum was validated are used extensively to inform the day-to-day content of the modules. It is recognized that issues of health promotion need to be centre stage and stressed frequently throughout the curriculum in a way that is clinically relevant and interactive (Ballas et al. 2000). *Choosing Health* (DoH 2004) is the Government's new White Paper on public health. In this document it is emphasized that there is a need to increase the numbers of health carers with experience of public health by strengthening public health in the training curriculum. Programmes of midwifery education are 'designed to prepare the student to practice safely and effectively so that, on registration, the student can assume the responsibilities and accountability for practice as a midwife' (NMC 2004, p. 30). The theme of health promotion is woven throughout the curriculum with the aim of defining standards that will enable childbearing women and babies to achieve optimum health and well-being (DoH 2003a). This is not achieved in isolation by the academic institute alone. The clinical placements and the midwives who mentor the students play a vital role in the preparation of the student.

PREPARING STUDENT MIDWIVES FOR THEIR HEALTH PROMOTION ROLE

It is important that student midwives consider their own ideas of health, in relation to both their own well-being and that of others. Students come with their own beliefs and values and this may have an effect on the way in which they learn and eventually practice (Ballas et al. 2000). Self-awareness is an element that needs to be fostered. It is a fundamental part of a health curriculum for students to explore their personal health values, their belief in the role of the profession for which they are training, and to consider the concept of being a role model. A health professional who leads what may be deemed an 'unhealthy' lifestyle (e.g. a smoker or living on take-away meals) may find it more difficult to provide health information (Conroy et al. 2004). Just attendance at a course related to health may raise self-awareness and create changes in lifestyle and attitude. However, attitudes are not easy to define because they have cognitive, affective and behavioural elements, and are also influenced by the values and beliefs held by the individual. Self-awareness and attitudes are areas explored within the midwifery programme and revolve around the students' own attitudes to health, their awareness of their own health behaviours and also their attitudes towards others' health behaviours. Attitudes may be strengthened through value clarification or changed through evidence and experience (Ballas et al. 2000). Ewles and Simnett (2003) suggest that opportunities should be provided to help students improve their own lifestyles and health. The Students' Union provides plenty of extracurricular activities and reduced rates to gyms, but the ability of many of our more mature students with families to take advantage is difficult to assess.

In the curriculum attitudes to other medical professions are challenged and the roles of different professions explored in an interprofessional module. The midwifery students look at interpersonal skills and ethics with seven other health-care groups, including medical, nursing, physiotherapy and pharmacy students. It is anticipated that, by meeting together and seeing how each profession trains and their different ways of working, will make working together, towards what is ultimately the same goals, easier to achieve on qualification. As the RCM (2003, p. 9) states 'a public health approach to midwifery would emphasise collaboration with a much wider group of professional experts'. This multiprofessional collaboration is also a recommendation in *Why Mothers Die* (Lewis and Drife 2004) and the NSF (DoH 2003a). This module moves towards meeting some of the education standards set out by the NMC (2004), which are:

> Provide seamless care, and where appropriate interventions in partnership with women and other care providers during the antenatal/postnatal periods. (pp. 37 and 39)

> Refer women who would benefit from the skills and knowledge of other individuals. (p. 38)

> Work collaboratively with other practitioners and agencies. (p. 44)

> Demonstrate effective working across professional boundaries and develop professional networks. (p. 46)

This module also works on raising the quality of interpersonal skills, concentrating particularly on communication. We encourage our students to explore communication in some depth and to become conscious of interactions between themselves and others in the clinical area. This includes other health professionals and, of course, clients and their families. The students also look at other ways in which information is conveyed, including an interprofessional critique of an information leaflet.

The mentor midwives are also involved with this because they are the ones who regularly see the students communicating with women. Allowing the student to practise and then provide feedback on performance is one of the most effective ways of acquiring effective communication skills (Cegala 2005). This helps the students to achieve the NMC competency on communication:

> Communicate effectively with women and their families throughout the pre-conception, antenatal, intrapartum and postnatal periods …
>
> (NMC 2004, p. 36)

Attitudes, self-awareness and prejudices are explored further in a module on sexual health. Midwives need specific knowledge and skills to be effective in meeting targets set in reducing sexually transmitted infections and the teenage pregnancy rate (DoH 2001, 2004). The NMC competencies (NMC 2004) mention provision of family planning and sexual health advice as skills required by students. However, discussion and promotion of sexual health and contraception have been shown to be a worry for student midwives (Bowden 2005). The module gives an opportunity for students to discuss their own beliefs about sex, relationships, sexual health and contraception in a safe and confidential environment. The expounding of myths and open discussion of issues has helped the students gain confidence to discuss sexual health with clients with the support of their mentors. This particular module is in the first year of training and the issues discussed are built on in different modules throughout the course. This module moves towards meeting one of the requirements of the midwife laid down in the *European Union Midwives Directive 80/155/EEC Article 4* (cited in NMC 2004) – 'To provide sound family planning information and advice'. It also endeavours to prepare the student on qualification to be ready to meet the health promotion requirements that are being asked for in the field of sexual health by different agencies already mentioned above, and to meet the issues raised in *Choosing Health* (DoH 2004).

The broader scope of the midwife's role is developed further in the module looking at the psychosocial context of midwifery. This module gives the student the opportunity to consider birth within the social context, exploring the diverse expectations of women and their families, and also exploring the social inequalities that may so adversely affect the health and well-being of a woman and her family. Acheson (1998) suggests that public health needs to be concentrated on society to bring about any change. Midwives have knowledge about the communities in which they work and the RCM advocates that midwives use this knowledge to become more involved with the choices being made in their communities (RCM 1999, 2001). This means moving away from the individual care and becoming population focused. Together with this comes a need for the health professional, in this case the midwife, to be more politically aware and for some to become more active in policy creation. Midwifery students need to learn how to empower women to become their own political voice. This module examines the role of the midwife in empowering women to identify their own needs and to speak for themselves. It also gives the student an opportunity to examine her own political/social beliefs and how they affect how they see the world and the women/families for whom they care. It is a time to challenge stereotypes, to reflect on prejudices and beliefs, and (hopefully) become more self-aware.

Of course we felt no curriculum would be complete without a module devoted to health promotion and public health. A requirement in the definition of a midwife adopted by the International Confederation of Midwives, the International Federation of Gynaecologists and Obstetricians and the World Health Organization (cited in NMC 2004, p. 33) is that a 'midwife has an important task in health counselling and education, not only for the women, but also within the family and the community'. This module also facilitates the student to meet the specific health promotion education standard set out by the NMC (2004, p. 42):

> ... contribute to enhancing the health and social wellbeing of individuals and their communities.

In this module the students look at the theory and approaches of health promotion and public health. This begins to equip the student with the knowledge needed to assess needs, and participate in and evaluate health promotion activities. The diverse needs of women, health inequalities and the needs of the family within the context of promoting health are explored in detail. Examination of the policy documents that affect the role of the midwife in relation to health promotion raises students' political awareness, which is necessary so that they can on qualification navigate the different health policy arenas (Whitehead 2003).

All the documents mentioned above influence the content of the course. It gives the students an opportunity to examine a specific health issue within the community with which they are working. This may be anything from aqua-natal to smoking cessation groups. The student looks at the chosen health intervention that is in place, and then considers the needs assessments that were required to establish the relevance of that intervention in their area, at whom the health intervention is targeted, how that population has been reached, what partnership working is required, how these partnerships were set up, and the effectiveness of the intervention and how it is evaluated. The ability to analyse and understand the political, social, economic and environmental issues that affect women are essential skills for a midwife (Adams 2001).

The mental health of women is an extremely important element of health promotion in midwifery (see Chapter 13). There is a module on this topic that is based on the requirements laid out in the document *Into the Mainstream* (DoH 1999). The students are first asked to examine their own prejudices, fears and beliefs surrounding mental ill health, as well as the many myths that they may have heard. For many, this is a completely new area of health; for others it is an issue that may affect them personally through family members or their own lived experience. As with the sexual health module, strict ground rules allow the students to discuss and explore issues in a safe environment. The issues surrounding the promotion of mental health well-being, identification of the at-risk groups, referrals, and what treatments may be required are discussed. Students are encouraged to spend a day in the nearby mother and baby unit or to spend time with midwifery specialties that have a mental health focus in the areas in which they are working.

The assignment asks them to do a case study of a woman at risk of or affected by mental ill health. This assignment and the module content support the students in achieving many of the NMC competencies (NMC 2004), including:

- Diagnose pregnancy, assess and monitor women holistically throughout the pre-conception, antenatal, intrapartum and postnatal period through the use of a range of assessment methods and reach valid, reliable and comprehensive conclusions. (p. 36)
- Determine and provide programmes of care and support for women. (p. 37)
- Refer women who would benefit from the skills and knowledge of other individuals. (p. 38)
- Work in partnership with women and other care providers during the postnatal period to provide seamless care and interventions. (p. 39)
- Care for and monitor women during the puerperium, offering the necessary evidence-based advice and support regarding the baby and self-care. (p. 40)
- Work collaboratively with other practitioners and agencies. (p. 44)

Midwives cannot change the fortunes of others or address the whole public health agenda, but, if every midwife facilitated a small positive change in women's health behaviour, then from small beginnings mighty things may happen. The health promotion elements that are fed throughout one 'direct entry' 3-year diploma in midwifery course go some way to achieving the ability to help and support women and their families to make those choices. The finer detail of how health promotion is threaded through the curriculum could be a book in itself. Potentially, for each student this finer detail will vary slightly depending on placements, assessment topics chosen and areas of interest. The high profile of health promotion helps to equip the student to practise on qualification in a holistic manner.

SUMMARY OF KEY POINTS

- Health promotion is an essential element in the training curriculum of student midwives, with influences from Government papers being influential in maintaining momentum and quality of training in this area.
- The theory–practice link is achieved by the invaluable support of the midwife mentors of the students.
- The NMC (2004) competencies can be achieved only with the theory being linked to practice in a conscientious manner.
- Health promotion needs to be threaded throughout the curriculum so the student can appreciate how it is evident in and affects all areas of practice.

REFERENCES

Acheson D (1998) *Independent Inquiry into Inequalities in Health*. London: The Stationery Office.

Adams L (2001) The role of health authorities in the promotion of health. In: Scriven A, Orme J (eds), *Health Promotion: Professional perspectives*, 2nd edn. Basingstoke: Palgrave, pp. 35–50.

Audit Commission (1997) *First Class Delivery. Improving maternity services*. Oxford: National Perinatal Epidemiology Unit.

Audit Commission (1998) *First Class Delivery: A national survey of women's views of maternity care*. Oxford: National Perinatal Epidemiology Unit.

Ballas PA, Asch SM, Wilkes M (2000) What students bring to medical school. Attitudes towards health promotion and prevention. *American Journal of Preventative Medicine* 18: 242–8.

Bowden J (2005) Sexual health awareness for midwifery practice. Unpublished work presented at Royal College of Nurses sexual health conference, February 2005.

Cegala D (2005) Interpersonal communication. In: Kerr J, Weitkunat, R, Moretti M (eds), *ABC of Behavior Change: A guide to successful disease prevention and health promotion*. Edinburgh: Elsevier, pp. 259–69.

Conroy MB, Delichatsias HK, Hafler JP, Rigotti NA (2004) Impact of a preventative medicine and nutrition curriculum for medical students. *American Journal of Preventative Medicine* 27: 77–80.

Department of Health (1993) *Changing Childbirth. Report of the expert maternity group*. London: HMSO.

Department of Health (1997) *The New NHS: Modern and dependable*. London: HMSO.

Department of Health (1998) *A First Class Service: Quality in the new NHS*. London: DoH.

Department of Health (1999) *Making a Difference: Strengthening the nursing and midwifery contribution to health and healthcare*. London: DoH.

Department of Health (2000) *The NHS Plan: A plan for investment, a plan for reform*. London: DoH.

Department of Health (2001) *The Nation Strategy for Sexual Health and HIV*. London: The Stationery Office.

Department of Health (2003a) *Getting the Right Start: National Service Framework for Children: Emerging findings*. London: The Stationery Office.

Department of Health (2003b) *Improvement, Expansion and Reform: The next three years priorities and planning framework 2003–2006*. London: The Stationery Office.

Department of Health (2004) *Choosing Health*. London: The Stationery Office.

Ewles L, Simnett I (2003) *Promoting Health: A practical guide*. Edinburgh: Baillière Tindall.

House of Commons Health Committee (1992) *Report on the Maternity Services*. London: HMSO.

Lewis D, Drife J (2004) *Confidential Enquiry into Maternal and Child Health 'Why Mothers Die'*, 6th report. London: RCOG.

Nursing and Midwifery Council (2004) *Requirements for Pre-registration Midwifery Programmes*. London: NMC.

Royal College of Midwives (1999) *Midwives and the New NHS. Paper 4: Public Health*. London: RCM.

Royal College of Midwives (2001) *The Midwife's Role in Public Health: Position Paper No. 24*. London: RCM.

Royal College of Midwives (2003) *Response to 'Securing good health for the whole population'*. London: RCM.

Royal College of Obstetrics and Gynaecology/Royal College of Midwives (1999) *Towards Safer Childbirth: Minimum standards for the organisation of labour wards*. London: RCOG.

UKCC Commission for Nursing and Midwifery Education (1999) *Fitness for Practice*. London: UKCC.

UKCC (2000) *Requirements for Pre-registration Midwifery Programmes*. London: UKCC.

Whitehead D (2003) The health-promoting nurse as a health policy career expert and entrepreneur. *Nurse Education Today* 23: 585–92.

9 PARTNERSHIP WORKING AND THE MIDWIFE

EDDIE WEST-BURNHAM

Much has been written on the links of poor health status, inequalities and material deprivation. As part of the present Government's attempt to address this issue, considerable focus has been placed on the benefits of partnership working; indeed it has become one of the 'fundamental principles' in delivering on the health inequalities agenda. With an emerging role in public health the midwife needs to develop an understanding of the concept of partnership working and the midwife's role within it.

This concept of partnership working is not a new one, but as far as current policy development is concerned it has emerged from being taken for granted and largely in the background to taking centre stage. So although it may be considered de rigueur by those writing public health policies, strategies and guidelines, what it means, how it works and how successful it could be can provide a considerable challenge to those health professionals, including midwives, who are charged with working with the concept.

The aims of this chapter are to identify what partnership working is, to explore how it works and to consider some of the challenges likely to be encountered. Some questions are offered for consideration together with opportunities for reflective practice within the framework of contemporary midwifery practice.

There are many different terms used to define partnership working. It is also referred to as joint working, alliance working and collaborative working, as well as interagency, interprofessional working and many more besides. However, for this chapter the term 'partnership working' is used throughout.

Reflection – 1

Before reading this chapter take some time to think about what you think partnership working is and how you see this as part of your role as a midwife.

A BRIEF HISTORY OF PUBLIC HEALTH AND PARTNERSHIP WORKING

Public health is anticipatory, focusing on the prevention of illness rather than the provision of treatment and care. It is entrenched in the positive theory of health and is concerned with the promotion of health and social well-being in its widest sense (Baggott 2000). This need to improve and protect the health of a population has existed for millennia – the Romans' approach to sanitation is a brief example. The development of public health in the UK truly started in the nineteenth century following the Chadwick report after the cholera epidemics in 1842. This raised the issue of health problems being linked to poor housing and insanitary conditions (Baggott 2000). Although progress in this concept was slow for the next 100 years or so, it was the creation of the National Health Service (NHS) in 1948 and its subsequent numerous reorganizations that led to a revival in public health strategies from the 1970s onwards.

This revival was influenced by a number of documents published by the World Health Organization (WHO) during the 1970s and 1980s, which were influential in the development and thinking about health promotion and public health, the most significant being the Ottawa Charter (WHO 1986). This charter identified three broad strategies for working to promote health:

1. Advocacy: to ensure the creation of conditions favourable to health.
2. Enabling: through creating a supportive environment but also giving people the information and skills that they need to make healthy choices.
3. Mediation: between different groups to ensure the pursuit of health.

The opportunities for the midwife to use her health promotion skills within the first two strategies are clear. However, the focus of this chapter is on the third point – partnership working – it is here that there is a danger that midwives will be excluded as most partnership working is driven through primary care trusts (PCTs) and public health networks, where there is little formal contact with midwives.

As part of the commitment to *Health for All by the Year 2000* (WHO 1985) the WHO outlined a set of guiding principles with which to orientate health promotion work, including:

- equity
- empowerment
- community participation
- multisectoral collaboration
- emphasis on primary health.

The Jakarta Declaration (WHO 1997) built on this platform reinforcing the right to health and emphasizing that health is essential for social and economic development. A number of priorities have been highlighted for the twenty-first century, including: promotion of social responsibility for health, increased investment for health development, and consolidation and expansion of partnerships for health.

The suppression and eventual publication of the Black Report in 1981, and the emergence of the international agenda for health promotion, brought to the fore the need for closer working relationships to meet the growing emphasis being placed on public health. The recent publication of the public health White Paper, *Choosing Health: Making healthy choices easier* (Department of Health (DoH) 2004a), offers a great opportunity to make a profound sustained approach to improve the public health of the population.

Equally there have been a number of recent publications that have identified the important role that midwives have within public health. In 2001 the Royal College of Midwives (RCM) in *Modernising Maternity Care* and the DoH in their *Midwifery Action Plan* clearly identified that midwives were ideally placed to work with women and their families across whole communities, to improve health and contribute to the reduction of health inequalities (DoH 2001a, RCM 2001). Key national policies – *Making a Difference* (DoH 1999a), *Saving Lives: Our healthier nation* (DoH 1999b) – have further identified an increasing public health focus for midwifery to strengthen the public health agenda. The most significant confirmation of the midwife's role in public health and in partnership working can be found in the *National Service Framework for Children, Young People and Maternity Services* where enhancing partnership is a principal aim (DoH 2004b). The success of midwifery partnership projects within the Sure-Start and Sure-Start Plus programmes, such as the safer sex enterprise in Powys, Wales (Lewis 2004), offer a strong practical example of all these policy recommendations regarding the midwife's role in public health.

THE CONCEPT OF PARTNERSHIP WORKING

Partnership working is about a collective response, in this instance to provide a unified effort to address health inequalities. This concept of a collective response can be challenging for agencies to embrace wholeheartedly because it requires a 'letting go' of power and control. Individuals and communities have a right to good health (here we have to accept the limitations of this chapter to discuss and deconstruct the meaning of rights). To facilitate this requires an understanding of social justice, promoting social inclusion, addressing poverty, promoting emotional intelligence and developing social capital. Accepting that many of these factors are essentially contested concepts and subject to many cultural, political and academic influences, it is hardly surprising that developing partnership working is at times so problematic.

Much has been written on what makes for a good partnership, Funnell et al. (1995) outline a number of different features for the success of partnership working, including:

- Commitment to the shared goals of the partnership
- Community involvement in all partnership activities
- Communication where partners share relevant information
- Partnership with equal ownership and appropriate input from each partner.

Guidance produced by the Improvement and Development Agency (2000) identified a range of skills required by councillors in local councils who were involved in developing and sustaining partnership working, the elements of which included:

- facilitating discussion between partners
- listening
- building consensus
- a commitment to providing resources
- building trust
- enabling and empowering others

- joint decision-making
- conflict handling and influencing skills.

To help tie all of this together, Moss Kanter (1994) offers a number of key elements that support and enhance the likelihood of a partnership maintaining its sustainability.

Important

The partnership must be seen as important to the participants, linked to their strategic objectives and long-term goals.

Investment

The partnership must be viewed as an investment, requiring time and resources. Benefits and costs should be seen as reasonably equitable over the long run.

Interdependence

The partnership must be based on mutual interdependence, recognizing that the members can achieve together what none could achieve alone.

Individual

Each member must display individual excellence and bring value to the collective enterprise.

Integration

There must be integration of purpose, vision and activity.

Information

Open, frequent and candid exchange of information is centred on effective collaboration.

Institutionalized

The partnership must be institutionalized, permeating the infrastructure of the participating organizations.

Integrity

Interaction among the members must be characterized by integrity and by relationships based on trust, commitment, honesty and good faith.

There are a number of other key elements that can make or break a partnership, including: the power differential and relationship maintained between the partners, the preservation of core values and identity, and the maintenance of mutual respect, trust and transparency.

On reviewing these key elements with the identified role of the midwife in public health, as mentioned in the national policies cited earlier in this chapter, it is quite clear that there are very few that would prove too difficult for midwives working within their current sphere of practice to achieve, if they wish to become more involved in partnership working. The only identifiable challenges would be knowledge about the actual structure and format of partnership working, which may be limited (Bennett et al. 2001, Hillier and Caan 2002), and overcoming the danger of midwives becoming excluded from the PCTs and public health networks from which local health improvement strategies are instigated (Edwards et al. 2005).

STRUCTURE AND FORMAT OF PARTNERSHIPS

Partnership working is now one of the fundamental principles underpinning the public health and health promotion philosophy in the UK and delivering the public health and health promotion strategy locally (Elston and Fulop 2002, Wildridge 2004).

This local delivery is in the shape of health improvement and modernization plans (HIMPs). HIMPs are 3-year local health strategies produced by partnership working. These partnerships are formed of a wide range of stakeholders from within and beyond the health service, they are driven by the local health authorities and feed into the local strategic partnerships (LSPs). LSPs were originally proposed as part of the neighbourhood renewal strategy (Social Exclusion Unit: cited in Ballach and Taylor 2001, p. 4) with a view to addressing the pace and proliferation of partnerships: 'stretching agencies, service users and communities to their limits.' The primary aims of HIMPs and LSPs are to improve the health and balance out the inequalities in health, social care and health provision of the local population (Elston and Fulop 2002).

Most partnerships work on a three-tier structure formed of a board or reference group that provides the strategic direction, a steering or programme group that examines how best to integrate policy and action and working groups based around both local priorities and localities. The working groups put the plans into action (Elston and Fulop 2002). Midwives would fit very well in the final tier with their knowledge and expertise of working with women, their families and the communities within which these families live. These working groups would provide midwives with an opportunity to experience working in partnership and provide a stepping stone to enter the other tiers as their knowledge and experience expand.

Membership of these partnerships is formed from representatives from many areas, including PCTs, hospital trusts, public health networks, local councils, community groups, police, voluntary organizations, the private sector and interested individuals from the public. From available evidence there seems to be few representatives from midwifery in these partnerships (Freudenstein and Yates 2001, Elston and Fulop 2002). Within the guidance over membership, there appears to be no maximum or minimum number of representatives to provide a quorum or allotted figure of how many from each represented area are allowed, on which to base equity (El Ansari et al. 2002, Elston and Fulop 2002, DoH 2005).

Although it is now an essential tenet of the Government's health agenda, partnership working is itself a contested concept. Rather like health, it means different things to different people at different times. Despite frequent requests for its use within national policies, the Government has provided no clear definition or guidance standards as to the format or structure of partnerships or partnership working, which leads to considerable flexibility.

This lack of Government guidance and the potential to be a 'movable feast' in terms of a definition – depending on who is defining it at the time – leaves the very term 'partnership' in danger of becoming a buzz word that has no clear meaning beyond being a 'nice' alternative to the long-tried and tested forms of governance (Rowe and Devanney 2003). Yet failure to understand the complexities that are inherent in the very nature of partnership poses serious dilemmas for those engaged in such schemes.

PARTNERSHIP WORKING AND SOCIAL CAPITAL

The principles of social capital have been around for some time; however, it is only since the publication of *Bowling Alone* (Putnam 1993a) that the term has been introduced to the broader vocabulary. Putnam himself describes it as 'features of social organisations, such as networks, norms and trust that facilitate action and cooperation for mutual benefit' (Putnam 1993b, p. 169). The term has since been popularized and, according to Woolcock (1998, p. 196), 'adapted indiscriminately, adopted uncritically and applied imprecisely'. Social capital has been described as an expansive concept: 'one that includes facets such as sociability, social networks, trust, reciprocity, and community and civic engagement' (Morgan and Swann 2004, p. 2). Putnam broadens this to include an individual's sense of belonging to a community, including positive participation in community activities. The development of social capital as a resource is related to the health, wealth and well-being of communities (Putnam 1993a). However, it would be wrong to think of social capital purely as a resource; it can also be seen as an explicit process that enables people and organizations to come together and work for reciprocal social benefit. Within health promotion its relevance is in its building of networks of communication – a factor that is fundamental to partnership working (Gillies 1998). Those working in health promotion, including midwives, will realize that individuals or communities are unlikely to change their behaviour unless it can be seen as both relevant and likely to result in some benefit. The same is true of those involved in partnership working.

Partnership working therefore fits the concept of social capital in several ways. It engages the social network of the communities: facilitates communication, and invokes trust, reciprocity and civic engagement (Gillies 1998). Midwives can look to developing social health gain by encouraging and sustaining the promotion of social networks and social capital, aided by their experiences of working within communities (Piper 2005).

If social capital in partnership working is to realize its potential there needs to be much greater importance placed on bringing together all those involved in public health to approve mutually agreed goals, a positive example of this being the national target for the reduction of inequalities in infant mortality (DoH 2001b). The report from The NHS Confederation (2003), outlining some of the outcomes from a conference on joined-up thinking in public health, gives a number of important actions that can be adopted to achieve this target:

- Building on Sure Start to improve early years' support in disadvantaged areas
- Reducing smoking in pregnancy
- Preventing teenage pregnancy and tackling its causes and effects
- Improvements in housing conditions for children in disadvantaged areas.

It will be apparent how the public health role of the midwife can contribute significantly to addressing these particular issues. The report also cites other forms of early intervention for the NHS, e.g. to increase immunization rates and breastfeeding, and to improve diet, family support and education about infant sleeping positions. All of these offer the midwife opportunities to enhance her role as a health promoter.

BENEFITS TO PARTNERSHIP WORKING

As Ballach and Taylor (2001, p. 1) observe: 'Superficially, partnership working makes a lot of sense.' Partnerships are a dynamic entity and as such the expectations and relationships are constantly evolving in a manner similar to that of the group. Establishing and maintaining a partnership is a complex, challenging process requiring commitment, patience, tolerance, trust, respect, a healthy dose of pragmatism and practical understanding. The success, or otherwise, of a partnership depends as much on the investment, commitment skills and attitude of the individual as on the engagement of the individual's host agency and the structure/environment in which the relationship exists.

This opportunity for successful collaboration needs to be built, as Nutbeam and Harris (2004) acknowledge, on the foundations of necessity and opportunity. The question is: Is the contribution being made by midwives to the public health agenda reaching its full potential? And indeed are midwives being allowed to realize that potential? Edwards et al. (2005) think not citing lack of formal contact between midwives and public health partnerships as one of the reasons for this.

Any organization that invests in its relationships and partnerships is much more likely to be seen in a positive light by those with whom it is working. As Field (2003) tells us in his outline of social capital, 'relationships matter'. He goes on to suggest that 'by making connections with one another, and keeping things going over time, people are able to work together to achieve things that they either could not achieve by themselves or could only achieve with great difficulty' (Field 2003, p. 1). If midwives are to realize their potential in partnership working and public health, it is important for them to engage fully with those involved at all levels of strategic development and to get involved at the community level.

Effective public health must be based on the WHO principles promoting upstream health interventions to prevent the development of avoidable ill-health rather than the traditional focus on downstream medical intervention that often treats preventable diseases. Public health requires action at all levels of the policy continuum and any health-care or social care professional working to a public health 'brief' has to subscribe to partnership working. Working across a health economy, public health practitioners (and by that is meant any individual working to improve the public's health) need to join with other key stakeholders, in housing, education, police, youth services and environmental health. The role of the midwife offers a unique opportunity to identify some of those individuals who are experiencing health inequalities and who are most vulnerable to any number of physical, social or psychological problems. However, at present they are not always best placed to feed these needs into any local strategy because they are outside the relevant networks.

There are a number of health promotion-related initiatives that all rely heavily on the success of partnerships within a social capital framework (Kawachi et al. 1999). Numerous opportunities exist in the health-promoting role of the midwife to develop partnership working. Two particular areas are highlighted here: promoting breastfeeding and reducing the prevalence of smoking in pregnancy.

Promoting breastfeeding has many physical and psychosocial benefits for both mother and child, including lowering the incidence and severity of many infections and protection from many adverse health outcomes (UNICEF 2004). There are numerous opportunities to promote breastfeeding that go beyond the normal exposure that the midwife will have with the mother. By taking a partnership approach to offering continuous psychosocial and emotional support before the birth, during labour and in the months after, both professionals and appropriately trained and supported laypeople could assist the mother and promote the benefits of breastfeeding.

It has been well documented that smoking has many potential problems for the woman, the fetus and neonate, including raised blood pressure, reduced birthweight and increased risk of sudden infant death syndrome (Twigg et al. 2004). In the *Independent Inquiry into Inequalities in Health*, Acheson (1998) offers considerable evidence to suggest how a decrease in prevalence in smoking during pregnancy is followed by a decrease in women who smoke after pregnancy, with the obvious benefits to the mother, child and those sharing her home. Any professional who has worked with people attempting to quit smoking will be aware of the difficulties encountered by all parties; however, pregnancy is a prime opportunity to encourage women who smoke to give up (Health Education Authority 1994) and a good opportunity for the midwife to work in partnership with other agencies, especially the smoking cessation services. It is therefore essential that those responsible for the care of both mother and child be linked into LSPs and other relevant systems.

The Health Development Agency (HDA) compendium *Tackling Health Inequalities* (DoH 2003) offers 35 examples of projects tackling health inequalities in communities across England. The range of projects is considerable with examples including: practical parenting courses in Andover, which encourages families to feel positive about their ability to parent; promoting perinatal mental health in Lincolnshire, which aims to reduce the incidence and impact of postnatal depression by working with parents before and after childbirth; and a scheme to tackle teenage pregnancy at Queen Elizabeth Hospital in London. This final programme aimed to improve teenagers' access to midwifery services and outcomes for newborn babies by developing maternity services that meet the specific needs of teenage mothers. The aim of the compendium was to feature 'snapshots' of projects tackling health inequalities in communities across England. There are a number of recurring themes common to meet projects; uppermost among these is the emphasis placed on partnership working. Key points or 'learning points' highlighted include the following:

- Get people and partners on board as soon as possible
- Give feedback to people and partners
- Develop partnerships: effective partnership working is when everyone knows where they fit into the picture.

CHALLENGES OF PARTNERSHIP WORKING

Activity – 1

Identify the challenges you see yourself facing when given the chance to work in a partnership.

Across the public health/health promotion agenda, the effectiveness of partnership working is often questioned by practitioners struggling to make the leap from theory ('it seems like it should be a good idea') to the reality of practice ('that worked well'). I am sure that many practitioners struggling with numerous competing priorities and ever-increasing workloads would agree with Brown et al. (2004) that, although the perceived wisdom is that joint working must be beneficial, there is, even at this stage, little evidence to support the notion.

If a manager of a busy midwifery unit is experiencing the considerable challenges of recruitment and retention, it is unlikely that setting up a partnership meeting to discuss how to meet targets for health inequalities is top of the agenda. It is easy to see how partnership working gets marginalized when priorities revolve around issues such as how to access resources, securing ownership of shared goals and overcoming the lack of mutual understanding between organizations, often with very different organizational cultures. Within any health organization there are likely to be difficulties when attempting to address the multitude of competing agendas, especially in an environment dominated by economic restraint and when decisions are often taken with the medical model taking centre stage. Indeed when considering the challenging area of evaluation, partnership working does not lend itself well to what has been described as the 'gold standard' of evaluation, the randomized controlled trial (RCT), the method most preferred by the medical establishment.

Partnership working is not the panacea to addressing the organizational, structural and strategic inadequacies when attempting to address health inequalities. Indeed, despite the widespread support for integrated community care in the UK, inter-disciplinary working between health and Social Services staff remains complex and tentative (King 2003), and unlikely to achieve sustained success unless it is given greater emphasis. This is especially true in relation to the unmet potential that the midwife has to contribute to partnerships and public health.

Considerable human and financial resources are devoted to the success of partnership working, yet many tensions, conflicts and challenges are encountered by all of those trying to forge the perfect partnership. Achieving consensus about the significance of a partnership is challenging, not least because, although many will subscribe to the principles of partnership working, following through with the necessary commitment is less easy to achieve. One of the potential pitfalls when implementing a partnership initiative is the potential disinvestment that a worker may experience should she or he become disconnected or detached from the process, and in the extra work needed in delivering relationships with outside organizations. Ownership of the process is therefore key as is clarity, of both purpose and method of delivery. This is where the concept of social capital in relation to organization development and partnership working becomes clearer.

It is important for midwives at all levels to engage in this process; to do so will require midwives to adopt what Edwards et al. (2005, p. 48) refer to as 'a radical and openly social stance to health'. This works very well when taking a broad approach to tackling health inequalities but has to be considered alongside Furber's (2000, p. 314) opinion that when looking at midwives' attitudes to health promotion:

> The patterns of views towards health promotion approaches were complex as midwives stated that they preferred societal approaches but worked in approaches that were focused on the individual.

It takes time to build trust in any relationship (professional or otherwise). The current often-unwritten policy of 'short termism' does not allow for relationships to grow and therefore does not facilitate healthy partnerships. Just as an individual or agency needs time to develop resilience in a new environment or to work in a new way, so partnerships need time to embed themselves into the psyche of local structures. This need for a more human approach to partnership working requires a cultural shift in the structural development and organizational management.

Relationships between statutory health and social care services and the voluntary sector have their roots in past practices and separate agendas and, as Andrews et al. (2003) recognize, partnership working does not emerge from a policy or service vacuum. In the study by Andrews et al. it was indicated that any partnership between the statutory and voluntary sectors in delivering packages of intermediate care would inevitably encounter challenges associated with multi-level, multi-professional and multi-agency collaboration. All of this takes place against a rapidly changing policy backdrop, where health providers and Social Services departments in England are attempting to develop partnerships in order to provide services effectively (Coleman and Rummery 2003).

All too often commissioners of programmes in health, community development, etc. are placed in a position where they are expecting agencies or partnerships to deliver solutions to complex health/social problems with limited resources, which are available for a fixed point of time (usually 1 year, occasionally 2, rarely 3 or more). We then ask for comprehensive evaluations that detail the impact of an initiative, this in itself being physically impossible.

The esoteric nature of the medical establishment can be an exclusive arena in which, even when patients' self-help groups are allowed to enter, the different values, language, etc. can inhibit equitable partnership arrangements. What is the solution? Look for the win–win scenario by using the principles and process behind a patient-focused approach. By embracing the concepts behind integrated care pathways and recognizing that the holistic reason for disease and illness require holistic solutions, an approach seen as positive by the medical establishment is much more likely to be successful than a process that is forced upon them.

Midwives play a significant role in reducing health inequalities and contributing to the public health agenda. The two areas of promoting breastfeeding and reducing the prevalence of smoking in pregnancy were indicated, but there are many others, especially in Sure-Start areas. In many areas of public health, professionals are still working in 'silos' where they remain isolated and disengaged from the broader public health debate. As Edwards et al. (2005, p. 48) have suggested, 'midwives are ideally placed to develop their public health role, but many feel isolated and unsupported in their personal development'.

SUMMARY OF KEY POINTS

- Midwifery is a profession already embedded in the ethos of public health. There is a broad professional consensus that maternity care should contribute to improving public health.
- Much has been written about the links between poor health status and material deprivation. As part of the present Government's attempt to address this issue,

partnership working has become one of the 'fundamental principles' in delivering on the agenda of health inequalities.

- There are many benefits to working in partnership, such as the opportunity for successful collaboration across various agencies to tackle the roots of health inequalities.
- The success of midwifery partnership projects within the Sure-Start and Sure-Start Plus programmes offer a strong practical example of the midwife's role in public health.
- The danger of midwives becoming excluded from PCTs and public health networks, from which local health improvement strategies are instigated, must be overcome.
- It is vital for midwives to realize their full potential in partnership working and public health, and it is important for them to engage fully with those involved at all levels of strategic development and to get involved at the community level.

REFERENCES

Acheson ED (1998) *Independent Inquiry into Inequalities in Health.* London: HMSO.

Andrews J, Manthorpe J, Watson R (2003) Intermediate care: the potential for partnership. *Quality in Ageing Policy Practice and Research* **4**: 13–21.

Baggott R (2000) *Public Health: Policy and politics.* Basingstoke: Macmillan Press.

Ballach S, Taylor M (2001) *Partnership Working: Policy and practice.* Bristol: The Policy Press.

Bennett N, Blundell J, Malpass L, Lavener T (2001) Midwives' views on redefining midwifery 2. *Public Health* **9**: 743–6.

Brown L, Tucker C, Domokos T (2004) Evaluating the impact of integrated health and social care teams on older people living in the community. *Health and Social Care in the Community* **11**: 85–94.

Coleman A, Rummery K (2003) Social services representation in primary care groups and trusts. *Journal of Interprofessional Care* **17**: 273–80.

Department of Health (1999a) *Making a Difference.* London: HMSO.

Department of Health (1999b) *Saving Lives: Our healthier nation.* London: HMSO.

Department of Health (2001a) *Making a Difference: Strengthening the nursing, midwifery and health visiting contribution. Midwifery Action Plan.* London: DoH.

Department of Health (2001b) *Tackling Health Inequalities: Consultation on a plan for delivery.* London: Department of Health.

Department of Health (2003) *The HDA Compendium Tackling Health Inequalities.* London: The Stationery Office.

Department of Health (2004a) *Choosing Health: Making healthier choices easier.* London: HMSO.

Department of Health (2004b) *Maternity Standard, National Service Framework for Children, Young People and Maternity Services.* London: The Stationery Office.

Department of Health (2005) *Creating Healthier Communities: A resource pack for local partnerships.* London: The Stationery Office.

Edwards G, Gordon U, Atherton J (2005) Network approach boosts midwives' public health role. *British Journal of Midwifery* **13**: 48–53.

El Ansari W, Phillips CJ, Zwi AB (2002) Narrowing the gap between academic professional wisdom and community lay knowledge: perceptions from partnerships. *Public Health* **116**: 151–9.

Elston J, Fulop N (2002) Perceptions of partnership. A documentary analysis of Health Improvement Programmes. *Public Health* **116**: 207–13.

Field J (2003) *Social Capital.* Routledge: London.

Freudenstein U, Yates B (2001) Public Health skills in primary care in South West England – a survey of training needs, obstacles and solutions. *Public Health* **115**: 407–11.

Funnel R, Oldfield K, Speller V (1995) *Towards Healthier Alliances.* London: Health Education Authority.

Furber C (2000) An exploration of midwives' attitudes to health promotion. *Midwifery* **16**: 314–22.

Gillies P (1998) Effectiveness of alliances and partnership for health promotion. *Health Promotion International* **13**: 99–120.

Health Education Authority (1994) *Smoking and Pregnancy: Guidance for purchasers and providers.* London: Health Education Authority.

Hillier D, Caan W (2002) Researching the public health role of the midwife. *British Journal of Midwifery* **10**: 545–7.

Improvement and Development Agency (2000) *A Councillor's Guide to Local Government.* London: HMSO.

Kawachi I, Kennedy B, Wilkinson R (1999) Crime: Social disorganisation and relative deprivation. *Social Science and Medicine* **48**: 719–31.

King N (2003) Professional identities and interprofessional relations: evaluation of collaborative community schemes. *Social Work in Health Care* **38**: 51–72.

Lewis M (2004) Working together to make a difference. *Midwives* **7**: 422–3.

Morgan A, Swann C (2004) *Social Capital for Health: Issues of definition, measurement and links to health.* HDA website: www.hda.nhs.uk (accessed April 2005).

Moss Kanter R (1994) Collaborative advantage: The art of alliances. *Harvard Business Review* July: 96–108.

NHS Confederation (2003) *Prevention is Better than Cure.* A report from a conference on joined-up thinking on public health. Nexus Report, Local Government Association and the Faculty of Public Health Medicine. London: NHS Confederation.

Nutbeam D, Harris E (2004) *Theory in a Nutshell, A practical guide to health promotion theories*, 2nd edn. Sydney: McGraw-Hill.

Piper S (2005) Health promotion: a framework for midwives. *British Journal of Midwifery* **13**: 284–8.

Putnam R (1993a) *Bowling Alone: The collapse and revival of American community.* New York: Simon & Schuster.

Putnam R (1993b) *Making Democracy Work: Civic traditions in modern Italy.* Princetown, NJ: Princetown University Press.

Rowe M, Devanney C (2003) Partnership and the governance of regeneration. *Critical Social Policy* **23**: 375–97.

Royal College of Midwives (2001) *Modernising Maternity Care: Commissioning for primary care trusts.* London: RCM.

Twigg L, Moon G, Walker S (2004) *The Smoking Epidemic in England.* London: HDA.

UNICEF (2004) *Health Benefits of Breastfeeding*: www.babyfreindly.org.uk/health.asp (accessed May 2005).

Wildridge V (2004) How to create successful partnerships – a review of the literature. *Health Information and Libraries Journal* **21**(suppl 1): 3–19.

Woolcock M (1998) Social Capital and Economic Development: toward a theoretical synthesis and policy framework. *Theory and Society* **27**: 151–208.

World Health Organization (1985) *Health for All by the Year 2000.* Geneva: WHO.

World Health Organization (1986) *The Ottawa Charter for Health Promotion.* Geneva: WHO.

World Health Organization (1997) *The Jakarta Declaration on Health Promotion into the 21st Century*. Geneva: WHO.

FURTHER READING

Baggott R (2000) *Public Health: Policy and politics*. Basingstoke: Macmillan Press.

Putnam R (1993) *Bowling Alone: The collapse and revival of American community*. New York: Simon & Schuster.

10 SEXUAL HEALTH PROMOTION IN MIDWIFERY PRACTICE

BEVERLEY BOGLE

Sexual health promotion requires social and political action, and educational and clinical interventions, which aim to improve the sexual health and well-being of individuals, families and communities. Despite Government commitment to this aim (Department of Health (DoH) 1992), the last 10 years has seen a rapid decline in the nation's sexual health. The National Strategy for Sexual Health and HIV (DoH 2001), and the Select Committee on Sexual Health (House of Commons 2003) provide alarming evidence supporting this view. Increases in sexual risk-taking behaviours, unintended pregnancies, abortions, HIV, Chlamydia and other sexually transmitted infections (STIs) have become a serious public health problem, now at crisis point and with escalating cost to the National Health Service (Alder 2003). Although sexual ill-health is widespread, it is more pervasive in vulnerable individuals and in people who suffer inequalities, e.g. women, teenagers, and black and ethnic minority people, especially those residing in inner city areas (DoH 2001, House of Commons 2003). Midwives are in an ideal position to improve the sexual and reproductive health of women. This can be achieved by working within targeted initiatives and developing health-promoting programmes that aim to enhance women's rational thoughts and sexual decision-making, restore their sexual self-esteem, and encourage sex-positive feelings, attitudes and behaviours.

In this chapter the concepts of sexual health and health promotion are clarified. Evidence is presented supporting the view that sexual health promotion is an integral facet to the midwife's role. Inherent challenges are explored, the need for midwives to encompass a broader and more holistic model of sexual health promotion discussed, and specific education required to effectively promote sexual health highlighted.

THE CONCEPT OF SEXUAL HEALTH

The concept of sexual health has stimulated debate in terms of definition clarity and operational coherence. To date there is no consensus on what this concept actually means. In 1975 the World Health Organization published the first definition, stating 'sexual health is the integration of somatic, emotional, intellectual and social aspects of sexual being in ways that are positively enriching and that enhance personality, communication and love' (WHO 1975, p. 6). This definition was criticized for its romantic positivism, because it omitted complex factors contributing to sexual ill-health. Critics also suggested, rightly or wrongly, that *love* was not a necessary ingredient for achieving sexual health. Since then there has been a plethora of definitions, varying in breadth, depth and complexity, all trying to capture this multifaceted phenomenon.

Activity – 1

Before reading further, take some time to write down what the concept of sexual health means to you.

Then, look at the two definitions below and consider how they differ from your concept.

> Sexual health is an important part of physical and mental health. It is a key part of our identity as human beings together with the fundamental human rights to privacy, a family life and living free from discrimination. Essential elements of good sexual health are equitable relationships and sexual fulfilment with access to information and services to avoid the risk of unintended pregnancy, illness or disease.
>
> DoH (2001, p. 7)

> Sexual health is a state of physical, emotional, mental and social well-being related to sexuality; it is not merely the absence of disease, dysfunction or infirmity. Sexual health requires a positive and respectful approach to sexuality and sexual relationships, as well as the possibility of having pleasurable and safe sexual experiences, free of coercion, discrimination and violence. For sexual health to be attained and maintained, the sexual rights of all persons must be respected, protected and fulfilled.
>
> WHO (2002, p. 1)

By reviewing these and other definitions, you will realize that, although there are similarities between them, they are fundamentally different. Definitions by their very nature are contextual, reflecting prevailing political and societal values when written, and are inclined to be utopian. This may limit their wholehearted acceptance and application in complex multicultural societies where sexual values and beliefs are constantly evolving and changing.

Definitions suggest that sexual health is personally defined and experienced, and can mean different things to different people. An individual's commitment to achieving and maintaining their sexual health is influenced by their world view and life experiences. Most people are likely to experience sexual ill-health at one time or another in their lives, so this idealistic state of well-being could be difficult to achieve and maintain. It is therefore easier to perceive sexual health as a non-static, fluctuating phenomenon, varying in degree of wellness and illness along a life-stage continuum. An individual's perception of her or his sexual health can move forwards or backwards along this continuum, at different times in life, depending on prevailing personal circumstances. It is important that individuals recognize and acknowledge their current position on the continuum, and take appropriate actions, if optimum sexual health is to be achieved and maintained. Definitions of sexual health also imply that it is a multidimensional concept, underpinned by many dynamic and changing entities that identify a person as a unique human being, including the following aspects.

Perceptions of self

An individual's perception of self, self-awareness and self-esteem can influence the choices made about how to live their life (Porritt 1990). Self-esteem, the evaluative component of self, can be high or low depending on circumstances, and is reflected in behaviours and interactions with others. An individual with low self-esteem may exhibit signs of anxiety, uncertainty, inferiority, insecurity, defensiveness, withdrawal, helplessness and dependency. He or she may lack trust in self and others, have difficulty dealing with anyone in authority and possess ineffective communicating skills (Engel 1995). The individual may even try to hide their low self-esteem when attempting to impress others by engaging in sexual risk-taking behaviours.

Expressions of sexuality

Sexuality is individually expressed throughout life in physical appearance, bodily movements, attitudes, behaviours, and sexual and non-sexual relationships. Expressions of sexuality are not static, varying at different life stages and underpinned by personal circumstances. There are many interacting dimensions of sexuality that underpin perceptions of sexual health, and at different times in one's life one or two dimensions may be given precedence (Figure 10.1). When expressed positively, it can bring much pleasure, but when expressed negatively it can cause physical and psychological harm (O'Driscoll 1998, Crouch 1999).

Sexual values and belief system

An individual's sexual values and beliefs are diverse and complex. They are governed by a value system that judges sexual activities as right or wrong. This self-imposed judgement can cause emotional dissonance when high expectations are unfulfilled, resulting in sexual ill-health. Mythical beliefs about sex and sexuality, e.g. 'sex in pregnancy will harm the baby', can increase anxiety and affect sexual functioning.

Sexual attitudes

Sexual attitudes are a reflection of an individual's sexual values and beliefs, influenced by their personality and social environments. A critical period of attitude formation is between the ages of 12 and 30 years (Crafter 1997). Once formed they are strong and resistant to change, and can be positively or negatively expressed. Attitudes formed during adolescent years can be precarious as personal identity is developed. Adolescents, while seeking independence, may engage in experimentation and sexual risk-taking behaviours resulting in STIs, unintended pregnancies and poor sexual health (Leishman 2004).

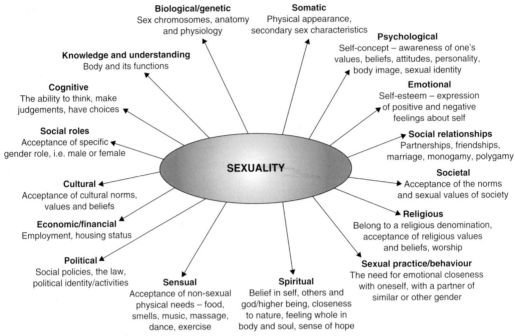

FIGURE 10.1 *Dimensions of sexuality (From Bogle 1996.)*

Sexual behaviours

An individual has the right to engage in sexual activities that are consensual, pleasurable and fulfilling, without causing physical or psychological harm. This is a basic human need and a human right (Maslow 1954, WHO 2002). Some individuals are vulnerable to sexual abuse as a result of their limited cognitive ability to make complex decisions or physical capacity to resist. Non-consensual sexual activities perceived as deviant can also impact on physical and psychological sexual health.

Perceptions of 'sex'

'Sex' is psychosomatic, involving all body senses, from which great pleasure is normally derived. It can mean different things to different people, but for the majority it is synonymous with 'sexual intercourse'. Some individuals may be unaware that sex can also include expressing and gaining sexual gratification in other sensual and non-genital ways that are equally pleasurable, e.g. sensate focus, visual and tactile stimuli. Therefore, perceived or actual failure in sexual acts and sexual functioning can cause considerable unhappiness, affecting their physical, psychological, social and spiritual well-being (Royal College of Nursing (RCN) 2000).

In summary, sexual health is a subjective and fluid state of well-being that is difficult to define, achieve or consistently sustain at optimum level. It is underpinned by an individual's perceptions of self, sexuality, sexual values and beliefs, sexual attitudes, behaviours and sexual knowledge. It should be holistic and positively enriching. Sexual ill-health is also subjective and, because the diagnosis is often dependent on self-referral, it can be difficult to identify, treat and monitor, particularly when the problem is psychosexual. Another salient feature of sexual ill-health is the associated strong negative emotions, e.g. increased anxiety, anger, hostility, fear, guilt, shame, blame and resentment. These emotions can be compounded by varying degrees of irrational thought, sexual risk-taking behaviour, low self-esteem, loss of confidence, loss of control, depression and sometimes suicidal tendencies (Bancroft 1989, Ingram-Fogel and Lauver 1990, De Silva 1994).

THE CONCEPT OF SEXUAL HEALTH PROMOTION

Sexual health promotion is the process of enabling people to increase control and improve their sexual health. To be effective it must be operational at both the macro- and the micro-levels within society and inclusive of all people. However, targeted initiatives can be aimed at people identified to be at high risk of sexual ill-health. A combination of interventionist strategies can be used (Box 10.1) that are underpinned by the principles of health promotion identified in *The Ottawa Charter for Health Promotion* (WHO 1986).

Box 10.1 Intervention strategies for sexual health promotion

Medical

- Promote medical interventions to prevent or ameliorate sexual ill-health
- Encourage people to seek early detection and treatment of sexual problems

Educational

- Give information and advice about causes and effects of sexual ill-health
- Explore myths, values and attitudes and enable informed decisions to be made
- Facilitate the development of skills required for healthy living

Behavioural

- Focus on client's attitudes and behaviour change to encourage adoption of healthier lifestyle to prevent sexual ill-health

Client centred

- Work with individuals on their own terms, addressing their sexual health issues, choices and actions
- Empower client to take responsibility for his or her own sexual health

Sociopolitical

- Action to change the physical environment to enable the choice of healthier lifestyle, by use of legislation, public pressure, lobbying, advocacy and community involvement

Naidoo and Wills (2000)

Sexual health promotion can be time-consuming and emotionally challenging, especially when working with individuals with perceived and/or actual lack of control over their lives. The difficulties they may have in making complex decisions, including changing their sexual attitudes and behaviours, are compounding factors. A multidisciplinary/multi-agency approach to sexual health promotion is, therefore, required, and midwives are key members of this team.

SEXUAL HEALTH PROMOTION AND THE MIDWIFE

Sexual health promotion is an important underlying principle of reproductive health (WHO 1998). Midwives, as lead professionals, are in a privileged position to make a difference to women's sexual health. During the maternity episode they develop relationships with women and their families and have the chance to gain valuable insight into the private sexual sphere of women's lives. This sexual health role is enshrined in statute. The Midwives rules and standards clearly outline that the midwife's activities should include 'preventative measures … and the extension of role to include gynaecology, family planning' (Nursing and Midwifery Council (NMC) 2004, p. 36). The European Union's Midwifery Directives endorse the midwife's role 'to provide sound family planning information and advice' (80/155/EEC Article 4, cited (NMC) 2004, p. 36). This sexual health role has been recognized by the Government and is explicit in several policy documents, e.g. antenatal testing for HIV (DoH 1999), initiation of discussion relating to sexual matters and sexual health assessment (National Institute for Clinical Excellence (NICE) 2003), and the extension of the Chlamydia screening programme to include pregnancy (DoH 2004).

Research and anecdotal evidence, regarding the sexual and reproductive health of women, illuminate midwives' professional responsibilities as primary care providers. The literature suggests that pregnancy and childbirth are common times when a couple's sexual relationship is most vulnerable. The physiological and psychological changes that occur impact on women's sexuality and sexual activity. Thus sexual problems are likely to occur. It is a time when altered body image can be perceived and felt by women, especially those who find it difficult to adjust to the normal physiological processes or whose reproductive organs are traumatized by childbirth (Price 1993, Clark 1997, Von Sydow 1999, Bartellas et al. 2000, Aston 2005).

Some women may not seek help for their sexual health concerns because of embarrassment in discussing personal and private matters. Some may feel that their problems are insufficiently important to justify requesting help, or that they are denied help through unavailability or inaccessibility. However, some women and their partners expect midwives to have professional knowledge and skills to address their sexual health concerns, and welcome opportunities to do so, despite their own feelings of discomfort and embarrassment in initiating discussions (Barclay et al. 1994, Victor and Barrett 1994). The implications of these findings are that midwives should be proactive in initiating discussions and not assume that all is well because a woman has not raised the subject herself.

Sexual health promotion by midwives is normally operational at the micro-level within society. Activities are facilitated individually or in small groups, using a variety of teaching and learning strategies that aim to give unbiased health-promoting information. Activities include anticipatory and amelioratory guidance that increases women's knowledge of normal processes of pregnancy and childbirth and the potential for sexual ill-health, giving women information and advice on sexual ill-health prevention, and providing appropriate care when sexual problems arise. Activities are traditionally underpinned by medical and educational strategies (see Box 10.1). Medical strategies tend to focus on prevention, identification and treatment of diseases, and trauma to the reproductive tract, e.g. STI screening in pregnancy, pelvic floor damage during labour, perineal healing postpartum, whilst educational strategies tend to focus on giving information and advice on a range of issues, e.g. healthy lifestyle and preparation for childbirth antenatally, and family planning/spacing and resumption of sexual activity postnatally.

CHALLENGES TO SEXUAL HEALTH PROMOTION

According to Curtis et al. (1995, p. 2) 'sexual health promotion includes any intervention that improves a patient's physical or psychological well-being … for example, contraception provision, cervical smears, safer sex advice, psychosexual counselling and other aspects of mental health'. In relation to this edict, one of the challenges that midwives face relates to the limited range of sexual health promotion activities that they currently engage in. They may perceive activities such as cervical smears, safer sex advice and psychosexual counselling, as suggested by Curtis et al. (1995), to be beyond their professional role.

A second challenge relates to the limited range and effectiveness of approaches to sexual health promotion that they currently use. The medical and educational approaches alone have a tendency to be fragmented and paternalistic, and have limited power in stimulating long-term changes in sexual attitudes and behaviours that are desired within society. Although it may be easier and less time-consuming to provide physical care, the importance of addressing the psychological causes and consequences of sexual ill-health cannot be overlooked. Individuals with sexual problems need extra time, help and support to restore, control and progress their state of sexual health along the continuum. Midwives may need to consider adapting other strategies that are client centred and facilitate change in formed attitudes and behaviours. This is pertinent in light of the growing public health concerns about the increasing prevalence of HIV and other STIs in pregnant women, the increasing incidence of domestic violence and abuse (Home Office 2003), and the disempowering emotional states associated with sexual ill-health (Bancroft 1989).

A third challenge relates to professional accountability. There has been no systematic evaluation to determine the effectiveness of sexual health promotion activities by midwives, with the exception of their well-established routine of giving postnatal contraception advice. However, the timing, quality, acceptability and cultural sensitivity of contraception advice and midwives' attitudes to this activity have been critically explored and challenged (Schott and Henley 1996, Smith et al. 2002, Hiller et al. 2003). There is also very little documentary evidence of the sexual health issues that midwives discuss with women, or the information and advice given on such matters. Although there may be legitimate concern regarding confidentiality of private and sensitive information shared, without clear documentation, the priority given to sexual health promotion activities, their quality and effectiveness cannot be monitored or assessed, nor improved communication between members of the multidisciplinary sexual health team facilitated.

A further challenge midwives face relates to personal and organizational perceptions of this role. Some midwives would argue that they do not have the time, knowledge or skills to engage in meaningful discussions with women about their sexual health concerns or to commit to providing comprehensive sexual health care. Some may surmise that, if a woman in their care has a sexual problem and wishes to discuss it, she would raise it herself, and therefore it is not within their professional role to enquire into a woman's private sexual life. Midwives may also view any wider involvement in sexual health promotion, beyond current antenatal screening, education for childbirth and the provision of family planning information and advice, to be an extension to their already demanding role, and feel there is little or no incentive. Ultimately they may believe a comprehensive and more holistic approach to sexual health promotion is the responsibility of other health-care professionals in other care settings, and nothing to do with them.

Some midwives may also view the lack of substantive guidance, from the Royal College of Midwives or employing NHS trust, on standards for efficient and effective sexual health promotion, as an indication of low professional accent. This view can be reinforced by lack of collegiate and managerial support (Bogle 1996). According to Burnard (1997) lack of clarity often brings anxiety and fear, leading to inaction. Some midwives may express discomfort with this sensitive and taboo subject. They fear 'opening up a can of worms', resulting in embarrassment, anxiety and inappropriate responses (Egan 2002). Discomfort leads to ambivalence, especially when midwives' personal sexual values and beliefs, attitudes and behaviours are incongruent with those presented by their clients. Challenges and barriers can be minimized with sensitive continuing education, agreed philosophy of care and vital clinical support.

KNOWLEDGE, ATTITUDES AND SKILLS FOR SEXUAL HEALTH PROMOTION IN MIDWIFERY PRACTICE

Some midwives may have specific knowledge and skills to provide holistic sexual health care. However, findings from the author's own research (Bogle 1996), and reflection seminars with midwives over the years, indicate that insufficient time is spent exploring the psychosexual aspect of sexual health.

A broader and more holistic philosophy of care at the micro-level is recommended, because effective functioning at this level is considered a prerequisite for macro-level activities. This philosophy should therefore support the view that an individual's sexual thoughts, feelings, attitudes and behaviour can underpin their unique expressions of sexuality and sexual health care needs. These dynamic entities are constantly evolving and subject to change, and should be periodically reviewed with women, even within one maternity episode. A model of care underpinning this view is presented in Figure 10.2.

To work within this model midwives need knowledge and understanding of female and male sexual anatomy and physiology, human psychosexual development, and the influence that psychological, sociocultural and sociopolitical processes have on sexual health. They also need specific attitudes, skills and confidence to discuss sexual matters without embarrassment, within professional boundaries, and knowing when and to whom to refer for expert therapy (O'Driscoll 1998). The education and skills development process could begin with the following prerequisites.

Enhanced knowledge of potential physical and psychosexual health concerns of pregnant women

The sexual health concerns of women are presented in Table 10.1. The list is not definitive, but gives insight into the numerous concerns women may have about their sexual health during maternity care. As can be seen, their concerns are both physiosexual and psychosexual. Problems may range in complexity and clinical presentation, and several may continue beyond the maternity episode. However, most problems can be anticipated and satisfactorily resolved with empathetic listening and meaningful discussions.

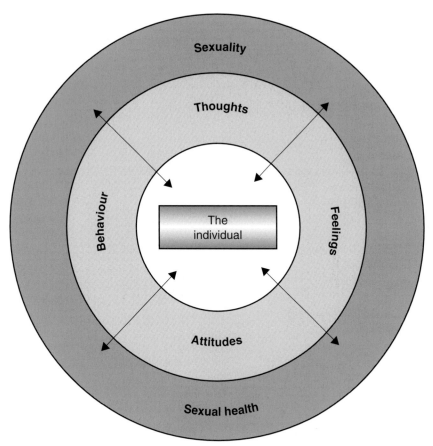

FIGURE 10.2   *Model of sexual health care. (From Bogle 1996.)*

Activity – 2

Before reading Table 10.1 make a list of the sexual health concerns that women may wish to discuss with you in your role as a midwife or student. Then review the list in Table 10.1 and identify topics that you would find challenging. Reflect on how you could deal with them.

Enhanced knowledge of rationale and manner in which women disclose their most intimate concerns

This awareness provides useful insights into a woman's psychological state. For most women, disclosure of a sexual problem is difficult, requiring courage and self-control. Some women may voluntarily disclose their sexual health concerns to a midwife, when feeling isolated or at crisis point, because they trust the midwife's professional knowledge and skills, and are respectful of the midwife's judgements and clinical decisions. Others may disclose their immediate sexual health concerns in a round-about way, sometimes pretending that the problem is their friend's, occurred in the past or is a possibility in the future. Disclosure may also be to vent feelings and emotions to anyone who will listen, to shock, seek sympathy or make social comparisons.

TABLE 10.1 *Examples of sexual health concerns of women during the period of midwifery care*

During antenatal care	During intrapartum care	During postpartum care
Body image	Vaginal examinations	Body image
Eating disorders	Vaginismus	Tiredness/fatigue
Subfertility treatment	Pain	Adjustment to motherhood
Unplanned/unwanted pregnancy	Body exposure	Variations in sexual desire and resuming sexual intercourse
Marital status, age, parity	Body fluids	breastfeeding
Miscarriage/abortion	Nipple stimulation	Milk ejection during orgasm
Variations in sexual desire and sexual activities in pregnancy	Instrumental vaginal delivery	Orgasmic pain
Sexual myths and values	Perineal trauma	Perineal discomfort
Lifestyle	Caesarean section	Vaginal size, discharge and dryness
Relationship discord/infidelity	Partner witnessing birth	Dyspareunia
Lesbian relationship	Family involvement	Contraception
Domestic violence	Female genital mutilation	Stress incontinence
Sexual abuse	Male attendants	Relationship discord
Antenatal screening for sexually transmitted infections (STIs)	Paternity	STIs
Female genital mutilation	Sex of baby	Condom use
Accommodation – space and privacy	Fear of death/stillbirth	
Occupation, e.g. sex industry	STIs	

The breadth, depth and truthfulness of sexual disclosures are influenced by the midwife–woman relationship. Age, gender, culture, religion, personality, social and professional status, of both woman and midwife, and the environment for disclosure all influence quality and reciprocity of information shared (Hargie et al. 1994). A woman may not feel that she knows or trusts the midwife to whom she is being asked to disclose. She may feel coerced if she has to divulge private and personal information to a stranger, fear judgemental unsympathetic treatment and have concerns that confidentiality will not be upheld. For some women, open, completely honest disclosures can take place in a short period of time, or slowly over several consultations, and be a relief when complete. Some women will use any opportunity to disclose and, if this happens in a public place, the midwife should respond to the here and now, without embarrassment. Reactions such as shock, disbelief, anger and repulsion, in the woman's presence, should be avoided. According to O'Driscoll (1998), negative reactions to a sexual problem can have a lasting and harmful effect on a woman's self-esteem and her intimate sexual relationship.

Enhanced self-awareness

This enables midwives to have positive regard and acceptance of women's sexual diversity and caring needs. Burnard (1999) also suggests that self-awareness enables individuals to discriminate between their own problems and those of others. Without conscious awareness midwives may identify too closely with women's sexual problems, imagining that they are similar to or the same as their own, or similar to other significant people in their lives. They may even project their own problems on to a woman, failing in their professional duty to focus on the woman's identified needs. Midwives should think carefully about what and how much of their own personal sexual life they share with a woman, in an effort to open up conversations, to express concerns for the woman's situation or to present a humane face.

Possessing sex-positive attitudes

Midwives need to consider their attitudes towards sex and sexual activities, in order to avoid judgemental and discriminatory practice. Respect and acceptance of the sexual values and beliefs that a woman holds are paramount to ensuring that sexual health promotion activities planned are congruent and acceptable. Sex should be viewed as a key element to a happy life, seen as a pleasurable experience and an effective form of communication between partners. Efforts should be made to encourage positive expressions of sexuality and sexual desire, and to raise women's sexual self-esteem. A midwife's sex-negative attitudes may manifest in stereotyping, stigma, prejudice and discrimination (Hayter 1996). Despite this, midwives also need to know that no one is free of judgemental thoughts and feelings, although some people may be more judgemental than others. As judgements about sexuality and sexual activities are particularly strong, some midwives may have difficulty repressing their own thoughts and feelings, and judgemental attitudes may be expressed. Inappropriate interpersonal communication can cause physical and psychological harm. Midwives can begin by acknowledging, accepting and respecting the strength of their personal judgements and regularly undertake self-review.

Ability to demonstrate genuine interest in a woman and her sexual problems

By demonstrating an empathetic approach, a midwife is able to put herself in the woman's shoes, genuinely feeling the way the woman is feeling about her problems. Although a certain amount of sympathy is required, Egan (2002) believes its usefulness is limited in helping. One of the dangers of being over-sympathetic is that the midwife can become immersed in the woman's self-pity, becoming her accomplice, and then begins to take sides with the woman without knowing the complete story. As guilt, blame and resentment often accompany sexual ill-health, midwives should be careful not to collude with a woman in apportioning blame, especially when directed at her sexual partner.

Ability to convey understanding in a language that the woman understands

Sexual language should be agreed, because vocabulary needs to be unambiguous. Medical and technical language should be avoided, as should language that may be perceived as judgemental. Bor and Watts (1993) suggest that health professionals should use clients' words and language to identify and acknowledge their sexual problems. The words women use to describe their sexual organs and sexual behaviours may be influenced by the context, the nature of the problem, maturity, sexual knowledge, cultural attitudes and interpersonal communication skills. Words used can be colloquial or technical, depending on with whom the individual is communicating. Sometimes a woman may use colloquial language inappropriately when communicating with a midwife, causing embarrassment. Midwives may need to explore colloquial words used by women primarily to identify words that are unfamiliar, uncomfortable to use and incomprehensible.

Ability to discuss a woman's feelings in a sensitive manner

Discussing a woman's feelings gives valuable insights into her emotional state. However, the midwife needs to be mindful that, in some cultures, people are brought up to believe that open display of emotions is unacceptable – talking about their feelings is considered to be a sign of weakness or self-indulgence. A tight upper lip is kept, fearing exposure to ridicule or loss of control. Burnard (1997) suggests that unexpressed emotions can distort thinking, and stop an individual from functioning fully or communicating feelings in words. By asking a woman how she feels about her sexual concerns a midwife can help her to express pent-up emotions. The midwife should pay particular attention to how the woman presents for the consultation, note and acknowledge the verbal and non-verbal feelings expressed, and sensitively confirm these with the woman.

Ability to discuss women's sexual relationships in a sensitive manner

Midwives routinely ask women about their relationships at the booking interview. The quality and honesty of responses will depend on how questions are asked. As relationships are value laden and particular types are deemed acceptable or unacceptable, the messages that a woman receives about her relationships from friends, family, health professionals and society are important to her. Some women may be concerned about the midwife's response if their sexual relationships fall below expectation. Midwives can sensitively ask a woman what she thinks as well as how she feels about her relationship. If the woman views her relationship as unsatisfactory, discussion can ensue on what actions she would like to take. This client-centred approach avoids giving information and advice prematurely, without knowing the bigger picture. However, when a child-protection issue is identified, the midwife should follow the guidelines for dealing with it (DoH 2003).

Ability to create an environment for open and effective communication

The importance of effective communication cannot be over-emphasized. This process begins at the initial antenatal booking interview when a comprehensive sexual health assessment is undertaken (Zawid 1994). Although there is no single approach or format, and personal style develops with experience, there are many guiding principles. NICE (2003) advises midwives to undertake sexual histories in an environment that is suitable for discussing sensitive issues. Sensitivity, privacy and confidentiality should be shown at all times, so a woman's sexual health concerns should never be discussed in the presence of anyone without the woman's express permission. The relationship between midwife and woman should be built on equality, trust and respect. Active and effective listening should be demonstrated because this leaves the woman feeling valued, acknowledged and validated (Porritt 1990, Stein-Parbury 2000).

Before assessment starts, the woman should be informed of the necessity of discussing personal and sensitive questions, and why complete and honest responses are necessary, e.g. to plan appropriate care. Reassurance of autonomy and control of pace and amount of information disclosed are important and the process should be unhurried. A prepared list of sexual health issues for discussion, proceeding from less

TABLE 10.2 *The PLISSIT model of sexual health intervention*

Give PERMISSION: convey willingness to discuss sexual thoughts and feelings. Provide assurance that concerns or practices are normal. Permission is often sufficient to resolve what may become a major problem

Offer LIMITED INFORMATION: provide information directly relevant to woman's concerns. Questions, sexual myths and misconceptions may be addressed. This can result in significant changes in sexual attitudes and behaviours

Make SPECIFIC SUGGESTIONS: provide specific instructions/suggestions to help woman change sexual behaviour to achieve/restore sexual health. The woman may need referral to an appropriate professional if knowledge and skills are lacking

Provide INTENSIVE THERAPY: provide highly individualized therapy, so referral to a specialist counsellor is necessary

Adapted from Annon (1974).

sensitive (medical and family history) to more sensitive questions, is recommended. Flexibility is essential, because questions may need to be adjusted according to responses. Questions should be universally phrased assuming everyone does everything, e.g. 'Many women are concerned about sexual activity in pregnancy, what might be your concerns?'. As already mentioned sexual language needs to be unambiguous, e.g. replace 'husband' or 'boyfriend' with 'sexual partner' and replace sexual intercourse with 'having sex'. Open-ended questions provide the opportunity for expressing thoughts and feelings. Questions beginning with 'how', 'when', 'what' and 'who' are appropriate, e.g. 'How has your pregnancy interfered with you being a sexual partner?'. Questions beginning with 'why' should be avoided, e.g. 'Why did you not go for counselling following your termination of pregnancy?'. Closed questions limit the range of responses, may be considered judgemental, and cause defensiveness, refusal to answer and return for consultation, or to be seen by that midwife again. At the end of assessment, the woman's priorities for sexual health care should be agreed and care planned accordingly.

Midwives may also wish to use a recognized framework to guide sexual health assessment. The PLISSIT model (Annon 1974) is highly recommended (Table 10.2). By using this systematic framework, midwives can develop their skills in opening up discussions with women and progressing a conversation in a meaningful and sensitive way. They soon become aware of the boundaries and limitations of their role and know when to refer women for intensive therapy (Ingram-Fogel and Lauver 1990, Zawid 1994, Alteneder and Hartzell 1997). Finally they could become adept in assisting women to identify, understand, accept and, where practical, overcome sexual problems. Ultimately this health-promoting process will help women to maintain some independence and control of their lives.

SUMMARY OF KEY POINTS

- Sexual health is multifaceted and difficult to define. It is a legitimate human right and midwives have a professional responsibility to enable its attainment.
- Sexual behaviour is a private and sensitive issue that some women may not wish to discuss with a midwife, who is perceived as a stranger.

- Private, confidential and comfortable environments facilitate initiation of discussions and open and honest disclosures of sexual health concerns relevant to women's actual or perceived needs. Acceptance and respect for individual uniqueness and right to self-determination should be shown at all times.
- Midwives should be self-aware, have knowledge of sexual phenomena, and know their limitations and referral pathways. Negative sex attitudes and unconcealed judgemental values and beliefs influence care provision and acceptance.
- Sexual health is a public health issue and midwives' role within the multidisciplinary team should be further acknowledged.
- Challenges and barriers to sexual health promotion can be overcome by sensitive education, collegiate and managerial support.

REFERENCES

Alder MW (2003) Sexual health – health of the nation: a decade later – a further failure. *Sexually Transmitted Infections* **79**: 85–7.

Alteneder R, Hartzell D (1997) Addressing couples' sexuality concerns during the childbearing period. Use of the PLISSIT Model. *Journal of Obstetrics, Gynaecology and Neonatal Nursing* **26**: 651–8.

Annon J (1974) *Behavioural Treatment of Sexual Problems: Brief therapy. 1.* New York: Harper and Row.

Aston G (2005) Sexuality during and after pregnancy. In: Andrews A (ed.), *Women's Sexual Health.* London: Elsevier Ltd.

Bancroft J (1989) *Human Sexuality and Its Problems.* London: Churchill Livingstone.

Barclay L, McDonald P, O'Loughlin J (1994) Sexuality and pregnancy – an interview study. *Australian and New Zealand Journal of Obstetrics and Gynaecology* **34**: 1–7.

Bartellas E, Crane J, Daley M (2000) Sexuality and sexual activity in pregnancy. *British Journal of Obstetrics and Gynecology* **107**: 964–8.

Bogle B (1996) An exploratory study of community midwives views, opinions and perceptions of their experiences in providing sexual health care. Unpublished MSc thesis, South Bank University.

Bor R, Watts M (1993) Talking to patients about sexual matters. *British Journal of Nursing* **2**: 657–61.

Burnard P (1997) *Know Yourself. Self awareness activities for midwives.* London: Chapman & Hall.

Burnard P (1999) *Counselling Skills for Health Professionals*, 3rd edn. London: Chapman & Hall.

Clark A (1997) Psychosexual disorders mini symposium. 5: Sexual problems and pregnancy issues. *Diplomate* **4**: 280–3.

Crafter H (1997) *Health Promotion in Midwifery. Principles and practice.* London: Arnold.

Crouch S (1999) Sexual health 1. Sexuality and nurses role in sexual health. *British Journal of Nursing* **8**: 601–6.

Curtis H, Hooligan T, Jewitt C (1995) *Sexual Health Promotion in General Practice.* Oxford: Radcliffe Medical Press.

De Silva P (1994) Psychological treatment of sexual problems. *International Review of Psychiatry* **6**: 163–73.

Department of Health (1992) *The Health of the Nation.* London: HMSO.

Department of Health (1999) *Reducing Mother to Baby Transmission of HIV. Health Service Circular 183.* London: NHS Executive.

Department of Health (2001) *The National Strategy for Sexual Health and HIV.* London: DoH.

Department of Health (2003) *What to Do if You're Worried A Child is Being Abused.* London: DoH.

Department of Health (2004) *Choosing Health.* London: DoH.

Egan G (2002) *The Skilled Helper*, 7th edn. Pacific Grove, CA: Brooks/Cole Publishing Co.

Engel B (1995) *Raising Your Sexual Self Esteem.* New York: Ballantine Books.

Hargie O, Saunders C, Dickenson D (1994) *Social Skills in Interpersonal Communication*, 3rd edn. London: Routledge.

Hayter M (1996) Is non-judgemental care possible in the context of nurses attitudes to patients' sexuality. *Journal of Advanced Nursing* 24: 662–6.

Hiller JE, Griffiths E, Jenner F (2003) *Education for Contraceptive Use by Women after Childbirth.* Cochrane Review, Cochrane Library issue 4. Chichester: John Wiley & Sons.

Home Office (2003) *Safety and Justice. The Government's proposal on domestic violence.* London: The Stationery Office.

House of Commons (2003) *Select Committee on Health. Third Report of session 2002/03 on sexual health.* London: The Stationery Office.

Ingram-Fogel C, Lauver D (1990) *Promoting Sexual Health.* Philadelphia: WB Saunders.

Leishman J (2004) Childhood and teenage pregnancies. *Nursing Standard* 18: 33–6.

Maslow A (1954) *Motivation and Personality*, 3rd edn. New York: Harper & Row.

Naidoo J, Wills J (2000) *Health Promotion. Foundations for practice.* London: Baillière Tindall.

Nelson-Jones R (2003) *Basic Counselling Skills.* London: Sage.

National Institute for Clinical Excellence (2003) *Guidelines for Antenatal Care.* London: NICE.

Nursing and Midwifery Council (2004) *Midwives Rules and Standards.* London: NMC.

O'Driscoll M (1998) Midwives discover sex. *The Practising Midwife* 1: 27–9.

Porrit L (1990) *Interaction Strategies*, 2nd edn. London: Churchill Livingstone.

Price A (1993) Altered body image in pregnancy and beyond. *British Journal of Midwifery* 1: 142–5.

Royal College of Nursing (2000) *Sexuality and Sexual Health in Nursing Practice.* London: RCN.

Schott J, Henley A (1996) Family planning considerations in multicultural society. *British Journal of Midwifery* 4: 400–3.

Smith KB, Van Der Spuy ZZ, Cheng L, Elton R, Glasier AF (2002) Is postpartum contraceptive advice given antenatally of value? *Contraception* 65: 237–43.

Stein-Parbury J (2000) *Patient as Person. Developing interpersonal skills in nursing.* London: Harcourt.

Victor C, Barrett G (1994) Is there sex after childbirth? *New Generation* 13: 24–5.

Von Sydow K (1999) Sexuality during pregnancy and after childbirth: A metacontent analysis of 59 studies. *Journal of Psychosomatic Research* 47: 27–49.

World Health Organization (1975) *Education and Treatment in Human Sexuality: The training of health professionals.* Technical Report Series No. 572. Geneva: WHO: www2.hu-berlin.de/sexology/GESUND/ARCHIV/WHOR.HTM#N3 (accessed July 2005).

World Health Organization (1986) *The Ottawa Charter for Health Promotion:* www.who.int/hpr/NPH/docs/ottawa_charter_hp.pdf (accessed July 2005).

World Health Organization (1998) *Definition of Reproductive Sexual Health* – available online www.who.int (accessed March 2005).

World Health Organization (2002) *Definition of Sexual Health*: www.who.int/reproductive-health/gender/sexual_health.html#3 (accessed March 2005).

Zawid C (1994) *Sexual Health, A Nurse's Guide.* Albany, NY: Delmar Publishers Inc.

FURTHER READING

Department of Health (2001) *The National Strategy for Sexual Health and HIV*. London: DoH.

Department of Health (2002) *The National Strategy for Sexual Health and HIV: Implementation action plan*. London: DoH.

Department of Health (2003) *Effective Sexual Health Promotion. A toolkit for primary care trusts and others working in the field of promoting good sexual health and HIV prevention*. London: DoH.

Royal College of Midwives (2001) *Position Paper No. 24: The Midwife's Role in Public Health*. London: RCM.

11 PROMOTING BREASTFEEDING: WHAT WORKS?

LOUISE LONG

Breastfeeding is an emotive subject. It provokes mixed responses from both mothers and midwives. Although it is seen as a 'natural' choice to many, our society has become a bottle-feeding culture. Bottle-feeding babies with artificial milk is widespread despite the 'breast is best' message. This presents very difficult issues when considering health promotion. Is it as simple as preaching the 'breast is best' louder and in different ways? Or is the answer more complex? This chapter examines these questions, suggests ways in which health promotion can be more effective and reviews initiatives that have been shown to work.

To start addressing these questions the current trends in breastfeeding need to be examined. The most comprehensive way of doing this is to study the Infant Feeding 2000 *survey (Hamlyn et al. 2002). This provides insight into where health promotion provision needs to be targeted. After having established what these areas are, this chapter discusses the contribution made by the* UK Baby Friendly Initiative (BFI) *and then details four areas of clinical practice that research has shown to be effective in getting breastfeeding off to a good start.*

INFANT FEEDING 2000 SURVEY

This survey of infant-feeding practices (Hamlyn et al. 2002) is conducted on behalf of the Department of Health (DoH) for the whole of the UK. It provides data on the incidence, prevalence and duration of breastfeeding and other practices adopted by mothers in the early weeks, up to around 9 months after the baby's birth. The survey is carried out every 5 years, this being the sixth in the series.

TABLE 11.1 *Incidence of breastfeeding*

Area of the UK	Percentage
England and Wales	71
Scotland	63
Northern Ireland	54
UK total	69

The survey is based on an initial national representative sample of almost 9500 mother and baby pairs born in the UK during 2000 and makes interesting reading, providing some of the best insights available into breastfeeding trends. The findings need consideration before any appropriate health promotion response can be made.

The survey gives figures for the whole of the UK, and divides the UK into three sections: Scotland, Northern Ireland, and England and Wales.

Incidence of breastfeeding

The survey defines the incidence of breastfeeding as the proportion of babies who were breastfed initially (this is all babies who were ever put to the breast, even if this was only on one occasion) (Table 11.1).

Prevalence of breastfeeding

The findings paint a picture of what could be called the 'classic breastfeeding mother'. These mothers were likely to have been:

- breastfed themselves
- having their first baby
- from higher socioeconomic groups
- in full-time education beyond 18 years
- 30+ years old
- from an ethnic group (two in three white mothers breastfed at birth, compared with around eight to nine in ten of each ethnic minority group)
- living in London and the south east.

Duration of breastfeeding and effect of events around birth

The figures illuminate where health promotion resources and effort are really needed. What is shown is that, of all the mothers who start to breastfeed, the steepest decline in duration occurs over the first 2 weeks (the first 2–3 days being the most critical). These findings are a real concern for midwives because it is over this period of time that this group of professionals have the most contact with the mother.

Starting with 100 per cent of all the mothers who initiate breastfeeding in England and Wales, the percentages of those still breastfeeding at various times are as shown in Table 11.2.

The events surrounding birth and in hospital have a great impact on the mother and influence whether or not she continues to breastfeed (detailed in Hamlyn et al. 2000).

TABLE 11.2 *Duration of breastfeeding*

Time	Percentage
Birth	100
1 week	85 (a loss of 15%)
2 weeks	80 (a total loss of 20%)
6 weeks	65 (a total loss of 35%)
4 months	45 (a total loss of 55%)
6 months	34 (a total loss of 65%)

HEALTH PROMOTION: WHOM ARE WE TARGETING?

It would appear that both the *Infant Feeding 2000* survey (IFS) (Hamlyn et al. 2000) and the DoH (2004) report give rise to two target areas for health promotion:

1. Lower socioeconomic groups who are less likely to breastfeed
2. The group of women who intend to breastfeed initiate breastfeeding, but have ceased doing so by the end of the first or second week – the 'lost 20 per cent' (see above).

For breastfeeding trends to increase, health promotion resources and effort must include this second target area. It could be argued that this area should take precedence over the first if resources are limited because there would seem little point in 'persuading' more women to breastfeed (irrespective of from which socioeconomic group they come), and then for these women to join the 'lost 20 per cent' 2 weeks after they have given birth.

How can the 'lost 20 per cent' be reduced? What can be done to prevent women becoming part of the 'lost 20 per cent'? How can health promotion work with this group? To answer these questions, consideration needs to be given to how women join this group in terms of their experience of maternity care. The 'cascade' of what occurs is outlined in Figure 11.1.

The 'lost 20 per cent cascade' and becoming part of it

The well-motivated first-time mother (Lucy 'lost') presents at the maternity unit for her first 'booking' appointment; she receives leaflets and information on breastfeeding – with the midwife recommending it as the 'best' choice. Lucy has already decided that she would like to 'try' breastfeeding.

During pregnancy Lucy attends hospital classes with her husband and there is one session on infant feeding during which a video is shown; the benefits of breastfeeding and bra fitting are discussed. Lucy now stands at the top of the cascade (Figure 11.1).

Lucy goes into labour at term, which is long and slow, with an epidural, resulting in a normal birth of a baby boy, 3.2 kg. Soon after birth the midwife, 'cleans up', weighs and dresses the baby, and gives him to Lucy to cuddle. The labour ward is busy and, although the midwife attempts to help Lucy breastfeed her new son, he seems sleepy so she moves Lucy to the postnatal ward.

Lucy settles on to the postnatal ward with the baby asleep in the cot beside her. When he stirs about 2 hours later Lucy attempts to breastfeed him again. She feels under-confident and unsure, and asks for help from a busy midwife who says she will be back shortly. When the midwife returns the baby has settled again and does not appear to want to feed. Lucy has moved down to the next part of the cascade in Figure 11.1.

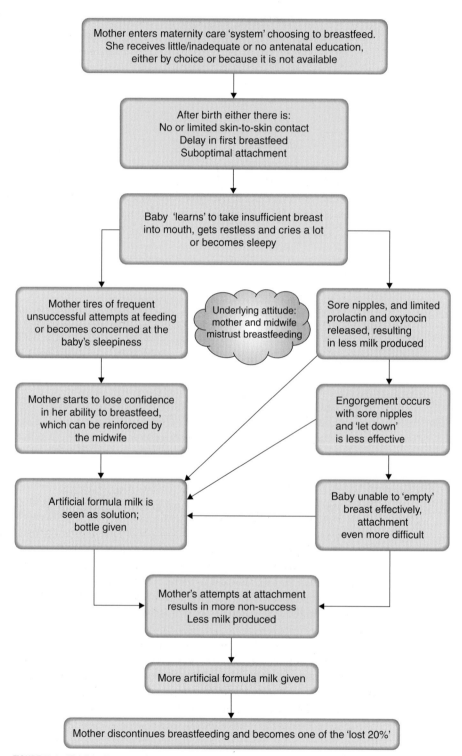

FIGURE 11.1 *The 'lost 20 per cent' cascade*

The day wears on. Eventually Lucy, concerned that her baby has not really had a feed yet, starts to lose confidence and may now start to see artificial formula milk as the solution. She approaches the midwife. What happens next is critical to this mother's breastfeeding – it hinges on the midwife's response. If either the mother or the midwife see giving artificial formula milk via a bottle as the solution, Lucy slides down the cascade much further, and without the intervention of skilled help is at risk of joining the 'lost 20 per cent'. If the midwife supports Lucy by building her confidence, showing her how to achieve correct attachment and encouraging skin-to-skin contact, it is still possible for breastfeeding to be initiated successfully.

This story and many similarly detailed stories occur regularly in maternity units. It shows the lottery of who joins the 'lost 20 per cent'. The midwife's role on the postnatal ward was more difficult as a result of Lucy's experience on the labour ward, which in turn was more difficult because of limited antenatal preparation, despite Lucy having attended classes.

Reflection – 1

Consider the Lucy 'lost' story and Figure 11.1.

- Do you think this could be the experience of mothers' care at your maternity unit?
- Reflect on what you may have done as a very busy midwife faced with Lucy asking for help.

Two issues emerge from Lucy's story and the 'lost 20 per cent' cascade that are key to mothers successfully initiating breastfeeding:

1. The attitude, knowledge and skill of midwives
2. Antenatal education, availability and content.

MIDWIVES, ATTITUDES, KNOWLEDGE AND SKILLS

Lucy's story highlights the need for the midwife to be a skilled practitioner. Ideally, this needs to start during pre-registration training so that, when qualifying, the midwife has the necessary knowledge and skills, and also understands how her attitude can affect practice. Once qualified, post-registration training needs to include regular updating.

There is currently no national curriculum for midwifery training. Each university develops its own course and then has this course validated by both the university and the professional body, the Nursing and Midwifery Council (NMC). Hence there is no national agreement about the knowledge and skills that need to be acquired during the pre-registration period. This has resulted in a haphazard skill acquisition during the training period and an inconsistency in newly qualified midwives' ability to support breastfeeding mothers. The clinical results of this are all too apparent in mothers' frequent complaints of inconsistent and conflicting advice. This works against a mother's own confidence and successful initiation of breastfeeding, damaging the credibility of midwives. These particular issues have been addressed by the UK BFI. This initiative has been evaluated to be effective, improving health-care professionals' ability to support women who are breastfeeding. It has now expanded its remit to include learning outcomes for pre-registration training involving midwives and health visitors (see below).

The UNICEF *UK Baby Friendly Initiative*

Before considering in detail some of the specific practices that have been shown to work in promoting breastfeeding, it is important to make reference to the BFI, which is described as:

> a global programme of UNICEF and the World Health Organization (WHO) which works with health services to improve practice. Health care facilities that adopt practices to support successful breastfeeding receive the prestigious UNICEF/WHO Baby Friendly award. In the UK, the BFI is commissioned by various parts of the health service to provide advice, support, training, networking, assessment and accreditation.

UNICEF (2000, p. 4)

To improve practice in hospital, the BFI has produced what it calls the 'Ten steps to successful breastfeeding', which can be seen in Box 11.1. These steps incorporate aspects of policy (step 1), in-service training (step 2), antenatal education (step 3), practice in postnatal care (steps 4–9) and working with other community organizations (step 10).

These steps and the award granted to maternity units that can demonstrate that they have implemented them have gained great credibility in midwifery. To date there are about 42 units in the UK with the award and others committed to working towards it. The award has been well evaluated and there is acknowledgement that it works (DoH 2004). One study shows that mothers are 28 per cent more likely to breastfeed in baby-friendly hospitals (Broadfoot et al. 2005).

Box 11.1   *The UNICEF* UK Baby Friendly Initiative: *ten steps*

All providers of maternity services should:

1. Have a written breastfeeding policy that is routinely communicated to all health-care staff
2. Train all health-care staff in the skills necessary to implement the breastfeeding policy
3. Inform all pregnant women about the benefits and management of breastfeeding
4. Help mothers initiate breastfeeding soon after birth
5. Show mothers how to breastfeed and how to maintain lactation even if they are separated from their babies
6. Give newborn infants no food or drink other than breast milk, unless medically indicated
7. Practise rooming in, allowing mothers and infants to remain together 24 hours a day
8. Encourage breastfeeding on demand
9. Give no artificial teats or dummies to breastfeeding infants
10. Foster the establishment of breastfeeding support groups and refer mothers to them on discharge from the hospital or clinic

World Health Organization (BFI – UNICEF 2000)

Activity – 1

Visit the BFI website at www.babyfriendly.org.uk and discover the following:

- Which is the nearest maternity unit to where you live that has 'baby-friendly' status?
- What does the website say is necessary in order for a maternity unit to gain a 'certificate of commitment'?
- What, in your opinion, is the key reason that prevents maternity units becoming 'baby friendly'?

Other than this work with maternity units and practice, the BFI has launched a new part of the initiative that involves best practice standards in the education of student midwives and health visitors. This involves all students having achieved a set of 19 learning outcomes by the end of their course of study; these are detailed on their website. Any university that can demonstrate that their students have achieved them will be granted an award. The award is likely to become as prestigious in education establishments as it is in maternity units, and it is hoped it will also go some way to establish basic minimum requirements in breastfeeding knowledge and skills in pre-registration education.

EFFECTIVE CLINICAL PRACTICES AND ANTENATAL EDUCATION

There is now a body of evidence to support several clinical aspects of practice. All of them interlink to prevent mothers from sliding down the 'lost 20 per cent' cascade (see Figure 11.1). They are:

- Mother and baby skin-to-skin contact and early initiation of breastfeeding (De Chateau and Wiberg 1977, Taylor et al. 1986, Thomson et al. 1997)
- Optimal positioning and attachment at the breast (Woolridge 1986, Righard and Alade 1992)
- Understanding baby's feeding cues and sleep states (Brazelton and Cramer 1991)
- The 'demand' feeding concept (Woolridge and Baum 1993, Wilde et al. 1995).

Undertaking any of these initiatives will make doing any of the others easier (Figure 11.2). All of these work towards successful initiation of breastfeeding and need to be incorporated into midwifery training and antenatal education.

For health promotion to be successful antenatal provision needs careful consideration. Classes need to be appropriate for the target group and assessable. They also need to build confidence and skills because this has been shown to increase breastfeeding rates. Their content needs to include the four points made above, particularly optimal positioning and attachment. This can be practised using dolls to give the mothers a 'feel' before the reality. There are videos that show the detail and benefits of skin-to-skin contact and the importance of the first early feed. Discussion can also take place with attitudes and beliefs about how often babies need to feed during the first few days. There is a useful exercise called 'the 24-hour clock' detailed in Schott and Priest (2002). This exercise encourages parents to consider the realities of the new baby and the effect on lifestyle. By including such exercises and making antenatal education more 'workshop' in style, parents can be more effectively prepared. For further resources, see the end of the chapter.

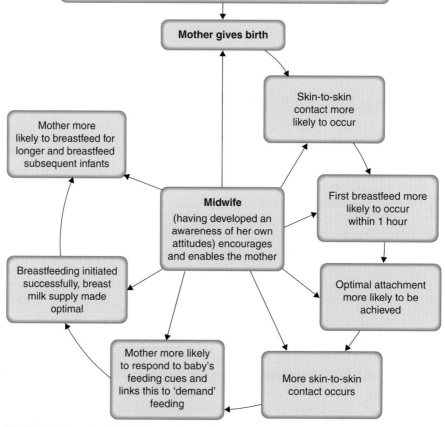

FIGURE 11.2 *Preventing the 'lost 20 per cent' cascade*

Activity – 2

Ask a female relative or friend, over retirement age, about their experience of feeding their baby/babies. You will often find that they are quite willing to talk! Questions you might include:

- What happened after the birth of your baby in hospital (or at home)?
- What was your experience of breastfeeding (if appropriate) like?
- How long did you breastfeed?
- When and why did you discontinue?
- Can you remember the advice midwives and/or health visitors gave you?
- Reflect on the answers you are given and how clinical practice today may be different.

MOTHER AND BABY SKIN-TO-SKIN CONTACT AND EARLY INITIATION OF BREASTFEEDING

In the last 5–10 years mother and baby skin-to-skin contact has gained a foothold in current midwifery practice. This change has been influenced by widely accepted research. It is hoped that it will become more and more commonplace with a positive effect on breastfeeding trends.

The concept is simple. The mother and baby stay together in skin-to-skin contact for periods of time. This ideally occurs at birth; after the baby emerges, he is lifted up to lie in between his mother's breasts. The mother and baby then remain this way undisturbed while routine practices such as weighing are delayed. The midwife gently dries the baby. A warm dry towel can be placed over them both if necessary. From this uninterrupted contact, it is hoped that the baby helps himself to his first feed, searching for the nipple. The mother or midwife may help him to achieve this – they may be surprised at his ability to do it himself.

Skin-to-skin contact has many advantages:

- Enhances the mother–baby relationship
- Encourages more natural and instinctive behaviour in both mother and baby
- Promotes breastfeeding
- Helps stabilize baby's temperature, respirations and heart rate
- Maintains baby's blood glucose levels.

Ideally all babies should be placed in skin-to-skin contact, not just after birth but also while being transferred to the postnatal ward. Any midwife receiving a baby on to a postnatal ward who is not in skin-to-skin contact with his mother could initiate it when helping the mother into bed. The earlier it is done the better and the greater the contribution to supporting breastfeeding.

OPTIMAL POSITIONING AND ATTACHMENT AT THE BREAST

Positioning is the term used to describe the posture and position of the mother and the baby in relation to each other. There are several variations but some common principles that must apply in all cases (Box 11.2).

Attachment is defined as the way in which the baby's mouth meets the mother's breast and therefore breastfeeds. Both positioning and attachment play a critical role in successful breastfeeding. When positioning is optimal, it paves the way for optimal attachment; if attachment is optimal, this triggers three important events.

The first is that the mother's nipples are less likely to become sore or cracked, thereby avoiding one of the main reasons mothers give for discontinuing breastfeeding. Second, the stimulation on the nipple and areola causes optimal prolactin and oxytocin release – so lactation is 'kicked' into action. These two hormones are crucial for all future milk production and release. Third, the breast is 'drained' or emptied effectively. This prevents engorgement and the 'feedback inhibitor of lactation' (FIL) factor operating adversely. This FIL factor is the name given to a protein in breast milk that can either increase or slow down milk production. If the breast becomes too full, it builds up to decrease milk and, if the breast milk is being removed effectively, the FIL levels fall so that the breast makes more milk.

FIGURE 11.3 *Various ways of positioning a baby for breastfeeding: (a) cradling; (b) cross-cradle; (c) 'football or rugby' hold; (d) lying down. Reproduced by kind permission of the WHO/UNICEF Baby Friendly Initiative.*

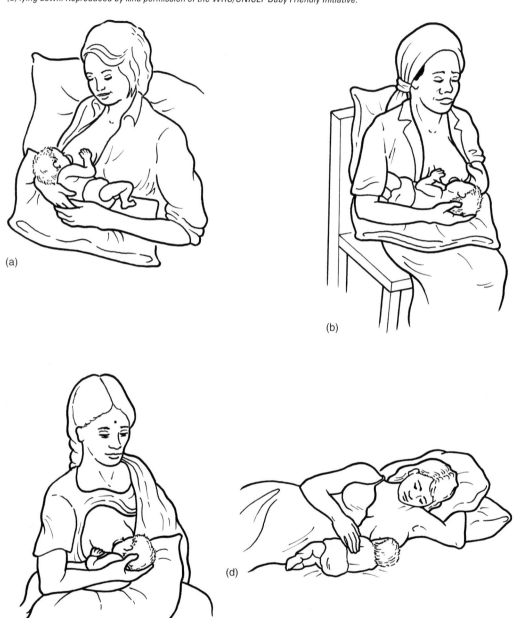

(a)

(b)

(c)

(d)

Without these three events occurring the mother is at risk of not optimizing her milk supply and discontinuing breastfeeding as a result of 'insufficient milk' (Renfrew et al. 2000). It is therefore imperative that midwives be not only aware of these factors but also fully competent at helping a mother secure optimal attachment and positioning.

Box 11.2 Principles of baby positioning

- Head and body in alignment, so the baby's neck is not turned at all
- Baby held close to the mother, without her leaning forward
- Nose should be opposite the mother's nipple
- Baby should be free to extend his or her head backwards
- Position should be sustainable
- A newborn baby should have his whole body supported, not just his head and shoulders
- Baby should not be too tightly wrapped

Adapted from WHO (1997)

Teaching positioning and attachment using dolls can be undertaken with student midwives during their training and with mothers during antenatal education. This can be quite easily included during a session, encouraging mothers to practise with the dolls and promoting discussion and interaction.

MOTHER AND INFANT POSITIONS

Cradling

Most mothers find this the most natural position to hold their baby (Figure 11.3a). The possible difficulties it causes with initial breastfeeding are threefold:

1. The baby is held to high in relation to the mother's nipple to achieve optimal attachment.
2. The mother has to help the baby attach with the crook of her arm and not her hand.
3. It can encourage the mother to lean forward instead of bringing the baby to her.

Cross-cradle

This position (Figure 11.3b) is ideal for the initiation of breastfeeding. It can overcome the problem of placing the baby too high or too low and gives the mother more control over the baby's head, shoulders and neck.

'Football or rugby' hold

This position (Figure 11.3c) is often used with newborns and provides a good alternative to cross-cradling. It can also be useful for mothers with large breasts.

Lying down

This is an obvious position for night feeding or after a caesarean section (Figure 11.3d). There are many variations that occur in regard to where the mother places her arm.

Whichever maternal position is used, there are seven key points to positioning the baby at the breast and these can be found in Figure 11.4.

Stages of achieving optimal attachment using a cross-cradle hold

Step 1 (Figure 11.4a)

The mother brings her arm around to hold her baby with his head and neck in alignment, close to her body, facing inwards, at the level of her nipple. Her hand should support the shoulders and neck but should not put any pressure on the back of the baby's head. He must have the freedom to move his head backwards and forwards. He should never feel 'forced' onto the breast.

Step 2 (Figure 11.4b)

The mother makes her breast a shape to fit the baby's open mouth. This can be done by making a 'V' shape with her thumb and fingers underneath her breast with her hand. The breast must not be lifted but held at its natural resting position, so that it will not drop when her hand is removed.

Some advisers dispute that the breast should be shaped at all.

Step 3 (Figure 11.4c)

When the baby opens his mouth wide, he needs to be brought towards the breast, aiming his nose at the nipple. The most important part of the breast to get into the baby's mouth is the areola, next to the baby's bottom jaw. Not achieving this is a major cause of sore nipples. Avoid leaning forward – note that the nipple goes in the baby's mouth just under the roof of his mouth, not centrally.

When optimal attachment is achieved, there will be more areola visible where the baby's nose is than where the baby's chin is – this can be shown to the mother.

If the baby is optimally attached, the nipple tip goes into the baby's mouth, reaches the baby's soft palate and the milk is ejected into the baby's throat. The nipple tip not

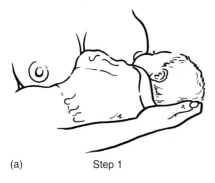

(a)   Step 1

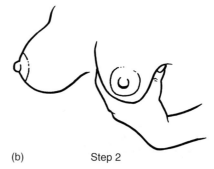

(b)   Step 2

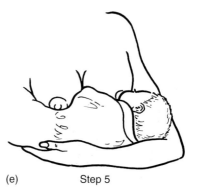

FIGURE 11.4 *Stages of achieving optimal attachment using a cross-cradle hold. (These attachment details have been adapted from Jamieson and Long (1997).)*

(e)   Step 5

being far enough into the baby's mouth, and moving against the baby's hard palate, is a major cause of sore nipples. This can be seen in clinical practice by the mother's nipple being 'flattened' out of shape when the baby comes off the breast.

Step 4 (Figure 11.4d)

The mother observes for signs of optimal attachment:

- There is no pain
- Mouth is open wide
- Rhythmic sucking with pauses
- Chin is against the breast
- If visible, more areola seen where the baby's nose is than at his chin.

Step 5 (Figure 11.4e)

When the signs of optimal attachment are present and the mother feels comfortable, she can gently let go of her breast and bring her arm around to the nappy, so that the baby is cradled in her arm with his head nestled in the crook of her arm at her elbow.

Note that women will vary in when they feel confident enough to let go of their breast. Some will take several feeds, others will take days.

Shoulders need to be relaxed down if they have risen up and the mother can lean back into the chair or pillows. It is now possible for the mother to have a drink or stroke her baby with her free hand.

Step 6 (Figure 11.4f)

If the baby is not well attached or if it hurts, the mother needs to slip her finger into his mouth, finding his bottom jaw, gently pressing down and easing him away. He must never be just pulled away or it will hurt as he tries to stay on.

The process can then be repeated after talking to the baby and asking him to open his mouth wide. It may take a few attempts in the early days while both mother and baby are learning.

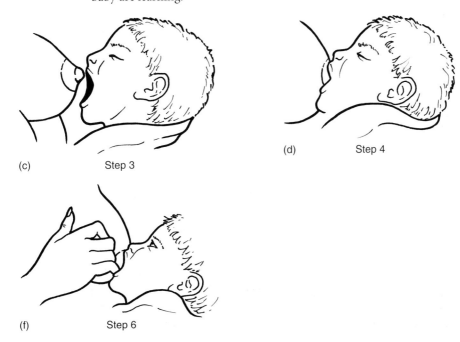

(c)   Step 3

(d)   Step 4

(f)   Step 6

Reflection – 2

Consider your own experience in clinical practice:

- Which position do you think mothers find is the easiest to adopt?
- Do you think most mothers need to 'shape' their breast to achieve optimum attachment in the first few days or not?
- What tips would you give a mother to encourage her baby to open his or her mouth wide?

THE 'DEMAND' FEEDING CONCEPT AND THE INFLUENCE OF ATTITUDES

An assumption can be made that midwives and mothers understand the concept of 'demand' feeding, and actually this is not always true – hence the different terms that have been used to try to describe it. 'Demand' feeding is perhaps the most common and the one the mother is most likely to use. However, the word 'demand' can sound pejorative and give the impression that the baby is 'demanding' from the mother and the mother has little choice but to respond to his 'demand'. In terms of enhancing the mother–baby relationship this may not be ideal. 'Baby led' or 'in response to baby's cues' are terms that have been used to convey the idea that it is the baby's behaviour rather than an imposed schedule that denotes when feeding occurs.

'Demand' feeding involves recognizing that the baby leads his own feeding by giving cues in his behaviour (e.g. awake and 'rooting') and that the mother responds to him by giving access to the breast. This means that breastfeeding is unrestricted in terms of either *frequency* (i.e. the number of times the baby is given access to the breast) or *duration* (i.e. the length of time the baby stays at the breast). So important is the 'demand'-feeding concept, that that BFI have included it as step 8 in their ten steps. Key to this concept working are several very important factors:

- The baby is 'normal' and his behaviour can be relied upon to give the necessary cues and thereby lead his own feeding.
- The mother understands and can recognize the baby's behaviour, which indicates that he wants to feed and then responds accordingly.
- The attitudes, values and beliefs of both the midwife and the mother are such that they trust the baby and the breasts to 'work'.

It is a good idea to consider the mother and baby as a 'pair', rather than individuals, because their relationship is so interrelated.

WHICH BABIES CAN BE RELIED UPON TO LEAD THEIR OWN FEEDING?

This is an important question and one that requires the midwife to make careful observation and assessment to answer. It is recommended that this decision is made with each mother and baby pair as soon after birth as possible and communicated to the mother as part of supporting her breastfeeding.

The following sets out guidelines using 'traffic lights' for the different categories:

- 'Green' relates to the majority of babies, whose behaviour can be relied upon to signal wanting to be fed. The mother simply needs to respond.

- 'Amber' relates to babies who may be less able in their behaviour to give feeding cues reliably. These mother and baby pairs need to be observed and assessed by the midwife over a period of hours before decisions can be made about whether they need any intervention. If well supported, these mothers and babies may not need intervention at all.

- 'Red' means that the baby cannot be 'left' reliably to lead his own feeding and will need intervention to establish breastfeeding.

'Green'

- Babies who are born at term (37–42 weeks)
- Babies whose weight falls between the 10th and 90th centile (a suitable centile chart can be seen in Johnston et al. 2003, p. 47)
- Babies whose Apgar scores are normal at 1 and 5 min (7 or above at 1 min and demonstrating increase at 5 min) and the following:
  - who were born by spontaneous vaginal birth, by uncomplicated 'lift out' forceps or ventouse, or by elective or emergency caesarean section
  - who may have had meconium-stained liquor (but normal Apgar scores, as above)
  - whose temperature has remained normal and stable (36.5–37.2°C) since birth
  - where there is no reason to suspect fetal infection
  - whose mother has not had pethidine (or any narcotic) drug during labour
  - who appeared 'normal' with 'normal' tone on first examination after birth.

'Amber'

- Babies who, although born at term (37–42 weeks), have weight between the 10th and 90th centile, but Apgar scores of 5 or 6 at 1 min after birth and needed intervention to establish breathing (irrespective of the mode of birth) or:
  - has an infection and needs antibiotics
  - whose mother has had pethidine (or any narcotics) in labour
  - who has had a more 'traumatic' forceps or ventouse birth.

Other babies in this category are given below.

Intrauterine growth restricted

This group need to have their behaviour observed carefully; they may well be able to lead their own feeding safely without intervention. Often they appear hungry and 'root' frantically for the breast, as if making up for lost weight gain *in utero*. If this is the case, although it may be tiring for the mother, these babies often initiate breastfeeding well. If not, the baby may well need intervention.

Born between 35 and 37 weeks' gestation

This group need individualized assessment of their sucking, rooting and swallowing reflexes before decisions can be made about the need for intervention and what form this may take (Lang 2002).

Pre-term babies who are returning to postnatal wards having spent time in the special care baby unit (SCBU)

This group have to be treated individually because their ability to breastfeed and developmental stage will vary. Hospitals have different policies concerning this practice.

Some congenital abnormalities

This group must also be assessed individually by an experienced midwife and neonatal medical team.

'Red'

- Babies who are above the 95th centile and/or whose mothers have diabetes
- Babies born before 35 weeks' gestation
- Babies born below the 10th centile or severely intrauterine growth restricted (IUGR)
- Babies who develop jaundice within 24 hours of birth (pathological)
- Babies with a diagnosed infection
- Babies with congenital abnormalities affecting any of the gastrointestinal tract and/or heart.

WHICH MOTHERS CAN RESPOND APPROPRIATELY TO THEIR BABY'S FEEDING CUES?

This is another important issue that needs careful consideration by the midwife. Some of these categories are more obvious than others. Mothers are more enabled to respond to their babies' feeding cues when:

- breastfeeding has been considered antenatally
- there is no separation between the two of them
- prolonged skin-to-skin contact is encouraged and a usual part of postnatal care
- the midwife is on hand to help support and encourage the mother to observe, interact and relate to the personhood of the baby.

Some mothers may find responding to their baby's feeding cues more difficult than others, usually because of physical or environmental reasons:

- Mothers who have had caesarean sections (this is a result of her restricted ability to move)
- Mothers who have had a general anaesthetic
- Mothers whose movement is still restricted as a result of the effects of epidural (or epidural tap) or spinal anaesthesia.

To assess the mother's ability to respond to her baby's feeding cues, the midwife needs to do so in the context of forming a relationship with her, however brief this may be, and observing how the mother is relating and responding to her baby. This provides insight into some of the mother's expectations and values. It may become apparent that the mother is unsure about how to recognize or interrupt aspects of her baby's behaviour, e.g. the mother may wait until the baby is crying before she attempts feeding and miss the 10 min before that when he is 'rooting' and attachment would have been easier. Another example would be a mother responding to her baby's 'rooting' or crying by letting him suck her finger instead of breastfeeding him, believing that he is not 'due' to be fed yet. The mother may want to impose a 'routine' limiting or restricting the *frequency* of the baby's access to the breast, or limiting the time the baby spends at the breast once attached. The midwife needs to work with the mother in observing the baby's behaviour and linking this to breastfeeding.

Reflection – 3

Consider the question: 'How easy is it to breastfeed?'

Now look at the line below. It represents a continuum ranging from 'very easy' to 'very difficult'. Place a mark that represents your own views:

Very easy   Very difficult

- Why do you think you put your mark where you did?
- What do you think this says about your beliefs about breastfeeding?
- How do you think these beliefs affect what you say to mothers?

Feeding cues and sleep states

Along with correct attachment, skin-to-skin contact and 'demand' feeding, it is important that the mother and the midwife have an understanding of feeding cues and sleep states. They involve the behaviour that the baby exhibits when becoming hungry and the different levels of consciousness he is in during sleep and awake time (Biancuzzo 2003).

By understanding and observation, mothers can breastfeed at the most appropriate time. Both 'demand' feeding and optimal attachment are thereby facilitated. The midwife can encourage the mother by pointing out to her the different behaviour as she is getting to know her baby. Figure 11.5 shows a summary of these six feeding cues and sleep states with the ideal breastfeeding times highlighted.

When helping a mother to initiate breastfeeding, the midwife needs to be aware that babies tend to be alert in the period immediately after birth and can then move into deep sleep. This is why skin-to-skin contact during this period is so beneficial to breastfeeding because the mother can become aware of her baby's behaviour. After this period of deep sleep, the baby's pattern can be highly individualized.

The following points should be noted when considering feeding cues and sleep states:

- Babies in deep sleep cannot breastfeed effectively and feeding should not be attempted. It should be noted here that sometimes mothers or midwives attempt to give a baby a bottle during deep sleep after trying unsuccessfully to attach him for breastfeeding. As milk will drip from a teat irrespective of sucking action on it, the milk will pool at the back of the baby's mouth. The baby then has three choices – either he swallows the milk, vomits it or inhales it. All three are undesirable and at best will undermine breastfeeding and at worst cause breathing problems.
- Pethidine (or any narcotic drug) in labour may hold a baby in deep sleep for longer. This needs explaining to the mother and she needs to observe any periods of light sleep or drowsiness and attempt stimulation. She will need to take every opportunity to feed her baby.
- The effect of epidurals on baby's feeding cues and sleep states is uncertain. Anecdotally, these babies can appear restless and move randomly from one state to another, making their behaviour more difficult to interpret and breastfeeding harder to initiate.
- Babies who are crying need to be consoled before feeding. This is because crying babies will bring their tongue up against the roof of their mouth. Unless the tongue is brought down attachment cannot be achieved.

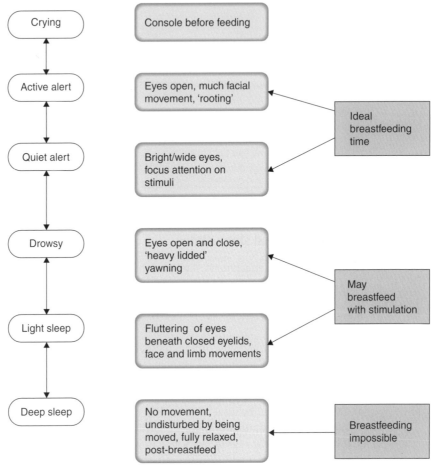

FIGURE 11.5 *Feeding cues and sleep states (assessing baby's readiness to breastfeed). (Adapted from Biancuzzo 2003 and Brazelton and Cramer 1991.)*

SUMMARY OF KEY POINTS

■ The *Infant Feeding 2000* survey (Hamlyn et al. 2002) provides the most comprehensive review of breastfeeding prevalence in the UK. It presents a picture of the 'classic breastfeeding mother' and details why women discontinue breastfeeding.

■ The *Baby Friendly Initiative* (BFI) has been shown to be an effective initiative in the promotion of breastfeeding.

■ The two target areas for health promotion are lower socioeconomic groups and women who initiate breastfeeding, but have ceased doing so by the end of the first or second week – the 'lost 20 per cent'.

■ There are four aspects of clinical practice that interlink to prevent women becoming one of the 'lost 20 per cent'. These are: mother and baby skin-to-skin contact, with early initiation of breastfeeding; optimal positioning and attachment at the breast; 'demand' or 'baby-led' feeding; and understanding the baby's feeding cues and sleep states.

REFERENCES

Biancuzzo M (2003) *Breastfeeding the Newborn*. St Louis, MO: Mosby.

Brazelton TB, Cramer BG (1991) *The Earliest Relationship*. London: Karnac Books.

Broadfoot M, Britten J, Tappin DM, MacKenzie, JM (2005) The baby friendly hospital initiative and breastfeeding rates in Scotland. *Archives of Disease in Childhood, Fetal Neonatal Edition* **90**: 114–16.

De Chateau P, Wiberg B (1977) Long-term effects on mother–infant behaviour of extra contact during the first hour post-partum: II. A follow-up at three months. *Acta Paediatrica Scandinavica* **66**: 145–51.

Department of Health (2004) *Good Practice and Innovation in Breastfeeding*. London: DoH.

Hamlyn B, Brooker S, Oleinikova K, Wands S (2002) *Infant Feeding 2000*. London: The Stationery Office.

Jamieson L, Long LM (1997) Promoting breastfeeding. In: Crafter H (ed.), *Health Promotion in Midwifery*. London: Arnold, pp. 201–77.

Johnston PGB, Flood K, Spinks K (2003) *The Newborn Child*. London: Churchill Livingstone.

Lang S (2002) *Breastfeeding Special Care Babies*. London: Baillière Tindall.

Renfew MJ, Woolridge MW, Ross McGill H (2000) *Enabling Women to Breastfeed*. London: The Stationery Office.

Righard L, Alade MO (1992) Sucking technique and its effect on success of breastfeeding. *Birth* **19**: 185–9.

Schott J, Priest J (2002) *Leading Antenatal Classes*. Oxford: Butterworth-Heinemann, p. 103.

Taylor PM, Maloni JA, Brown DR (1986) Early suckling and prolonged breastfeeding. *American Journal of Diseases of Children* **140**: 151–4.

Thomson ME, Hartstock TG, Larson C (1997) The importance of immediate postnatal contact: its effect on breastfeeding. *Canadian Family Physician* **25**: 1374–8.

UNICEF (2000) *The UNICEF UK Baby Friendly Initiative: A brief guide*. Geneva: UNICEF.

Wilde CJ, Prentice A, Peaker M (1995) Breastfeeding: matching supply with demand in human lactation. *Proceedings of the Nutrition Society* **54**: 401–6.

Woolridge M (1986) The 'anatomy' of infant sucking. *Midwifery* **2**: 164–71.

Woolridge M, Baum JD (1993) Recent advances in breastfeeding. *Acta Paediatrica Japonica* **35**: 1–12.

World Health Organization (1997) *Breastfeeding Management: A modular course*. Geneva: WHO.

World Health Organization (1998) *Evidence for the Ten Steps to Successful Breastfeeding*. Geneva: WHO.

FURTHER READING

General breastfeeding texts

Lawrence R (1999) *Breastfeeding*, 5th edn. St Louis, MO: Mosby.

Riordan J, Auerbach KG (1998) *Breastfeeding and Human Lactation*, 2nd edn. Boston, MA: Jones & Bartlett.

Royal College of Medicine (2002) *Successful Breastfeeding*, 3rd edn. London: Churchill Livingstone.

Examining the research base for care

Renfrew MJ, Woolridge MW, Ross McGill H (2000) *Enabling Women to Breastfeed*. London: The Stationery Office.

Correct attachment

Page LA (2000) Breastfeeding in caring for your baby. In: *The New Midwifery*. London: Churchill Livingstone, p. 369.

Woolridge M (1986) The 'anatomy' of infant sucking. *Midwifery* **2**: 164–71.

Woolridge MW (1986) Aetiology of sore nipples. *Midwifery* **2**: 172–6.

Sleep states and feeding cues

Cadwell K, Turner-Maffei C, O'Conner B, Blair A (2002) *Maternal and Infant Assessment for Breast Feeding and Human Lactation*. London. Jones & Bartlett Publishers Inc., pp. 38–40.

Biancuzzo M (2003) *Breastfeeding the Newborn*. St Louis, MO: Mosby, pp. 237–9.

'Demand' feeding

WHO/Child Health Development (1998) *Evidence for the Ten Steps to Successful Breastfeeding, Step 8*. Geneva: WHO, pp. 68–70 (available from the BFI website).

Skin-to-skin contact

Anderson CG, Moore E, Hepworth J, Bergman N (2003) Early skin-to-skin contact for mothers and their healthy newborn infants. *The Cochrane Database of Systematic Reviews* Issue 2 Art. No: CD003519.

Ashmore S (2001) Implementing skin-to-skin contact in the immediately postnatal period. *MIDIRS Midwifery Digest* **11**: 247–50.

FURTHER RESOURCES

Department of Health (2004) Infant Feeding and Child Nutrition Pack. This pack contains details of all DoH recommendations, a full directory of breastfeeding resources and details of good practice innovation in breastfeeding. Packs can be obtained free of charge from: DH Publications Orderline, tel: 08701 555455, or by emailing: dh@prolog.uk.com

All WHO/UNICEF Baby Friendly Initiative, available from their website: Babyfriendly.org.uk

Videos from 'Mark it television associates' website: www.mark-it-television.com

Titles include: *Infant Feeding Cues*; *A Guide to Successful Positioning*; *Dealing with Problems and Coping with the First Week*. Note: other videos are detailed in the DoH (2004) pack detailed above.

12 SMOKING, PREGNANCY AND THE MIDWIFE

MOYRA M HEGGIE

Midwives have a vital role in smoking cessation and pregnancy; they are a source of knowledge, and have the interaction skills to convey information about the benefits of quitting smoking for a woman, her partner and her family. Using a health promotion model, such as that of Prochaska and DiClemente (1984), can help a midwife identify the stage of change a woman may be in, and so adopt appropriate strategies to assist her. Knowing that her midwife is interested, supportive and encouraging can be a very positive aspect to a woman to stop smoking and continue as a non-smoker. The midwife also has an awareness of Government and local smoking cessation services and so is able to make seamless referrals for the woman to receive further help and support.

Smoking is becoming increasingly antisocial and is clearly acknowledged as being detrimental to the health of all who are exposed to it. Midwives are in a strong position to motivate and encourage better lifestyles in the childbearing population and should continue to develop their knowledge and skills to promote health in this arena. This chapter aims to provide knowledge about the effects of smoking and why women smoke, and some helpful strategies to achieve smoking cessation using an acknowledged, successful model.

GOVERNMENT POLICY AND TARGETS FOR SMOKING CESSATION

In the UK smoking causes 120 000 preventable illnesses each year, including a third of all perinatal deaths (Department of Health (DoH) 2004a). Just under half of the 10 million who smoke are women, 9 per cent of these being aged 11–15 years. Interestingly 69 per cent of all smokers say they want to stop (DoH 2000); if successful it would help improve their long-term health and reduce the estimated annual cost of £1.4–1.7 billion to the nation.

It is estimated that more than a third of women in the UK, under the age of 44 years and therefore potentially fertile, are currently smokers. The *National Service*

Framework for Children, Young People and Maternity Services (the NSF) (DoH 2004b) states that pregnant women and their partners who smoke should receive clear information about the risks of smoking as well as support from smoking cessation services such as the National Health Service's (NHS) Stop Smoking Service. Here possible preconception advice and support could be given as well as information about the risks of second-hand smoke or passive smoking. About one-third of perinatal deaths are attributed to smoking and this could be minimized if care were provided by integrated multidisciplinary and multi-agency teams (DoH 2004b).

The range of smokers varies geographically, but predominates in urban con-urbations and socially deprived wards (Twigg et al. 2004). Women, especially those from deprived areas, and schoolgirls are potential targets for additional resources. Numerous publications incorporating statistics and targets and setting out Government strategies can be accessed from Department of Health and linked websites, e.g. the Health Development Agency (HDA), now combined with the National Institute for Clinical Excellence (NICE) to become the National Institute for Health and Clinical Excellence (see Further reading). Many of these strategies set targets for smoking cessation.

Smoking cessation targets

- Reduce the rate of smoking from 32 per cent in 1998 to 26 per cent by 2010, with 800 000 smokers from all groups successfully quitting at the 4-week stage by 2006. This equates to 900 quitters per primary care trust (PCT) compared with 167 and 333 in 2001–2 and 2003–4, respectively.
- Update practice-based registers by March 2006 so that patients with coronary heart disease and diabetes receive appropriate advice and treatment on diet, physical activity and smoking, with a focus on those with hypertension and a body mass index >30.
- Reduce by 1 per cent per year the proportion of women smoking throughout pregnancy, especially those from disadvantaged groups, as part of the national target to reduce the mortality difference between different socioeconomic groups by at least 10 per cent by 2010, starting with children aged under 1 year. The Public Service Agreement (DoH 2004c) target is 21 per cent or fewer smokers by 2010, with the rate in manual groups at or below 26 per cent.

(Taken from DoH 2002; cited by West et al. 2003a, p. 7.)

To achieve Government targets of reducing smoking means that 4–5 per cent of smokers need to stop – a tall order especially where the levels are already quite low, e.g. Wokingham or Chiltern and south Bucks at 20 per cent compared with north Liverpool, north Manchester or eastern Hull at 40 per cent (Twigg et al. 2004). Increased referrals are needed by members of the primary care team, including midwives, who are a major source for clients' referral to specialist smoking cessation services (West et al. 2003b). The vital role of the midwife is to initiate the process of change, identify need and refer appropriately, and to provide continuing support, as women become non-smokers during their childbearing episode (West et al. 2003b).

SERVICE RECOMMENDATIONS

High-quality supportive care related to the individual needs of women and their babies is advocated by the NSF (DoH 2004b). Government targets demand an increasing level of success in smoking cessation, with what may be an increasingly intransigent core of smokers. Funding has enabled health promotion departments specially to train and update professionals to give the care and support to women (West et al. 2003b); these professionals can be part of the managed networks of maternity and neonatal care (DoH 2004c). However, the HDA recommends that PCTs continue to develop and permanently fund specialist smoking cessation services alone or in partnership with other PCTs, and when merging to retain existing key personnel. A full-time person, supported by core staff, should coordinate services, commission and organize training, act as a point of contact with midwives, other services and agencies, oversee monitoring and ensure that the service adapts to changing needs. PCTs need to develop comprehensive strategies to reach all smokers with a focus on low-income and pregnant smokers, as well as meeting the needs of ethnic minority populations and linking with acute hospital and mental health trusts (West et al. 2003b). These strategies will involve the maintenance and development of the smoking cessation skills of all health-care staff, links with local community groups and national tobacco control initiatives being made and maintained to promote referral and treatment services. Group treatment or individual face-to-face counselling is effective, but groups may be impractical in an area with a sparse population or limited transport.

Nicotine replacement therapies (NRT) and bupropion (Zyban) are an integral part of the treatment package offered; however, bupropion is not advised during pregnancy (NICE 2002). Pregnant women, if unable to otherwise quit, can use NRT (available as patches, microtabs and lozenges) instead of smoking. The possible risks to the fetus from NRT are less than those of continued smoking (West et al. 2003b). In a quasi-randomized experiment in Denmark NRT gum or patches produced a 13 per cent quit rate in 75 women 1 year after delivery (Hegaard et al. 2004). NRT is available at pharmacies or on prescription from general practitioners (GPs); smoking cessation specialists hope soon to be able to prescribe NRT. The drugs are given as part of an abstinent-contingent treatment, so clients must not smoke while using NRT. If planning to stop before conception women can be prescribed bupropion for 7–14 days before the quit day (NICE 2002), although contraception should be guaranteed during treatment. Partners should be encouraged to give up at the same time and can also be prescribed bupropion; together with special couple groups, this can raise success rates (Thompson et al. 2004).

The NSF proposes that women and their partners requesting support to stop smoking be provided with specialist services within managed care networks to improve children's health development and resilience to problems in later life (DoH 2004c). Smoking cessation midwives achieve higher quit rates compared with midwives providing holistic care, unless the latter are specially trained. In north Staffordshire one such group of midwives achieved quit rates of 13 per cent (West et al. 2003a). Attending training days run by the PCT or local higher education institution can provide midwives with the knowledge and skills to help and the opportunity to rehearse interactions with women. If women are not asked about their smoking, referrals to specialist midwives or smoking cessation specialists will not occur. Despite referral to the PCT smoking cessation department, many women fail to respond, and some may prefer the care from their named midwife, or require telephone prompts or home visits by the smoking cessation midwife, particularly if they have young children and find going out troublesome (West et al. 2003b). The primary midwife can help to support the women in her care to quit smoking. Women who do not engage at all or deny that they are smoking provide the midwife with a challenge. This is when the cessation training comes into its own.

Whatever the case, as mentioned earlier, the midwife needs first to identify women and their partners who may be ready to stop smoking. To achieve this goal, the midwife needs an insight into the effects of smoking and why people start and continue to smoke.

EFFECTS OF SMOKING TOBACCO

Cigarettes and cigarette smoke are potentially lethal to the smoker and those nearby; Box 12.1 lists the contents of cigarettes, and Boxes 12.2 and 12.3 give some of the possible effects to the smoker and others.

Box 12.1 Content of cigarettes

Mutagens and carcinogens
Butane
Cadmium
Phenol (carbolic acid)
Hydrogen sulphide
Formaldehyde
Hydrogen cyanide
Tar and derivatives – coat lungs
Carbon monoxide – creates carboxyhaemoglobin, limiting oxygen in blood
Nicotine – more addictive than heroin, absorbed in 7 seconds, causes vasoconstriction

(Raw et al. 1998, DoH 2000, Twigg et al. 2004)

Box 12.2 Physical effects of smoking

Related to women	Other effects
Reduced fertility	Platelet adhesion and rigidity of red blood cells
Delayed ovulation	Increases blood viscosity, increasing deep vein thrombosis
Spontaneous miscarriage	Increased endogenous opiates, adrenaline, noradrenaline,
Ectopic pregnancy	antidiuretic hormone, lung mucus, vessel permeability, plaque
Pre-term labour	formation and blood fatty acids
Placenta praevia	Dementia
Placental abruption	Gastrointestinal and respiratory system cancers and disease
Nicotine staining	Renal and bladder cancer
Osteoporosis	Myeloid leukaemia
Earlier menopause	Cardiovascular disease, especially stroke and myocardial
Prematurely aged skin	infarction
Carcinoma of cervix	More postoperative complications, especially after general
	anaesthesia

(Raw et al. 1998, DoH 2000, Twigg et al. 2004)

Box 12.3   Effects of passive smoking on babies and infants

Intrauterine growth restriction
Increased mortality
Sudden infant death syndrome
Meningitis
Glue ear
Lower education attainment
Leukaemia
Reduced lung:body ratio
Respiratory disease
More hospitalization
Smaller and lighter at 5 and 7 years
More visits to GPs
More likely to be a smoker

(Raw et al. 1998, DoH 2000, Twigg et al. 2004)

MOTIVATIONS AND DIFFICULTIES ENCOUNTERED BY SMOKERS

Many non-smokers find it hard to comprehend the compulsion to start or continue to smoke tobacco, especially considering the effects identified in Boxes 12.2 and 12.3. Initiation into smoking may be triggered by curiosity, peer pressure and being accepted in a social group. Young people are renowned for their antiauthoritarian stance; knowing that it is 'bad' makes it attractive. If parents smoke and there is no education to the contrary offspring will often follow the tradition. The possible appetite suppression and weight reduction combined with media coverage of idols who smoke give a sophisticated or macho aura, and make smoking attractive. For some, smoking is a form of stress relief; it is commonly associated with poverty, unemployment and a fatalistic outlook on life. Having a cigarette is a treat or reward, can enhance mood and confidence, calm or ease pain and may help concentration. The subsequent addiction and withdrawal problems then arise, but the habit, combined with the perceived enjoyment and comfort, means that many continue. Some may avoid trying to stop, fearing failure, because smoking cessation is recognized as seriously challenging (Hawkes 2004, Plowright 2004, Wetter et al. 2005).

Goddard and Higgins (2000) found that young people, especially girls, are more likely to start and continue smoking, a significant point in areas with high teenage pregnancy rates. Your local PCT or strategic health authority statistics can be identified via the HDA website for *The Smoking Epidemic in England* (www.hda.nhs.uk). Addressing the issues of adolescent smoking may be an area where midwives' public health role can extend by contributing to personal social health education in schools to counteract smoking triggers and provide general information about the effects of smoking in pregnancy (Markham et al. 2004).

ATTITUDES TOWARDS TOBACCO SMOKING

The media coverage of the Government White Paper, *Choosing Health: Making healthy choices easier* (DoH 2004d), illustrates arguments for and against the banning or restriction of smoking in public places. Comparisons are made with Scotland, Ireland and New York where bans have already been enforced. Supporters of a ban cite cases of lung cancer resulting from secondary or passive smoking and suggest that a partial ban is not enough (Roberts 2004); opponents consider the evidence insufficiently robust and claim that the economic and social effects will be negative. Some suggest that the Government is creating a nanny state with intrusion into every aspect of our lives to limit our eating, alcohol intake, gambling and smoking. The reader can access some of the arguments via websites for ASH (2004) and FOREST (2004) (see also Useful information and contacts). In this potentially confusing and authoritative context, midwives are required to raise awareness on health issues so that women and their partners can be supported to make lifestyle decisions to benefit their own health, the health of their family and that of the forthcoming baby.

To approach women in the right manner, we need to acknowledge our prejudices and try to suspend judgement. It is easy to say that everyone knows that smoking is harmful and anyone who smokes must be foolish. Are we all so perfect that we do nothing potentially harmful to our health? Ideally none of us would actively choose to behave in ways detrimental to our health, but human nature is such that at some time most of us have behaved inappropriately.

Reflection – 1

Examine your own life and identify a time when you have been tempted to act (or have acted) without full consideration of your health, e.g. eating poorly, driving too fast, not exercising, having unprotected sex, drinking to excess.
Make notes when considering these questions:

- Why did you do it?
- How did it make you feel?
- Did you think about the possible risks?
- Did you know what the risks were?
  - if yes why did you still do it?
  - if no would you still be tempted knowing it was possibly unsafe?

Think about your response to campaigns about your health-threatening activity?
If you cannot recall a situation that fits this reflection, perhaps someone you know has, so try imagining their responses to these questions or better still ask them!

When women who are planning to conceive or are pregnant tell us they smoke it can evoke many feelings. Maybe in light of the reflection we can rethink how 'foolish' or 'wrong' we feel they may be and consider more clearly the action that could be taken to help them stop smoking.

But what if the midwife smokes? Is she a hypocrite telling pregnant women to stop? Her defence may be that she is not pregnant. Perhaps she cannot raise the issue, so maybe we need to support her in quitting (Wiseman 2004). However, the midwife who is a former smoker can empathize, and appreciate the addiction and difficulty of quitting; she may have used many of her clients' arguments to justify not stopping, e.g. 'I will not be a drain on the state as I shan't live to draw my pension', 'Tax paid on cigarettes pays for the health care needed', 'My auntie/mother/father has smoked 30 a day since a teenager and is OK', 'My last baby weighed 7 lb', and can defuse their impact. The woman may be encouraged by the midwife's success in quitting and remaining a non-smoker, so strategies can be discussed more personally. The financial implications of smoking are another factor that non-smoking midwives find hard to accept when the family may be struggling to make ends meet, as is evident from the statistics linking social deprivation to substance misuse (DoH 2004c).

The non-smoking midwife needs an empathetic, not a critical judgemental approach to assisting her client; quitting is very difficult, so we need to adopt positive messages (Rew 2004). Consider the busy woman pregnant with her second or third baby, whose partner, family and peers smoke, and who feels that her only solace in a frantic day is to sit for a few minutes 'having a fag'. Maybe a carrot rather than a stick will help her; we can acknowledge the difficulties but encourage her that by feeling fitter she can be more active with her children, and dream how she can spend the money saved. Saying she smells like an ashtray or instilling even more guilt than she already feels will alienate some (Rew 2004) and scare-mongering tactics may encourage a defiant lighting up!

Activity – 1

Access the HDA website (www.hda.nhs.uk) and estimate the purchase costs and levels of dependence for a real or imagined client. See how much money she could spend on alternatives in a week, month or several years if she quit.

Additional costs highlighted by the midwife could include home decoration, air fresheners, laundry and housework, and more dental hygiene. These may be persuasive arguments for some people, but even so some women will forego their food to pay for their cigarettes.

Social isolation exists for smokers: they are increasingly ostracized as a danger to others' health and for their unpleasant odour. For some equating their smell with sitting next to someone with severe, stale, body odour on crowded public transport may be a revelation. Quitting may reactivate dormant friendships with non-smokers with the simultaneous exclusion from smoking peers and the loss of the camaraderie that they shared. It is hard for even the most enthusiastically supportive midwife to compete with some of the pressures, so sustaining the woman's non-smoking status needs active support from her partner and friends.

Motivation can be further encouraged by visual cues of damage with raised carbon monoxide levels in expired air, a falling lung expiratory capacity, a baby's bottle full of cigarette ends floating in tar, pictures of lungs impregnated with tar and smoke, and babies exhaling smoke. These may have some immediacy, whereas cancer rates and long-term debility seem remote when the smoker enjoys the habit now.

The presence of a pregnancy or planning a pregnancy may be sufficient motivation for the woman and her partner to stop smoking. For most smokers motivation is the key; once in place it provides the impetus to quit often helped by NRT. Once stopped, ex-smokers need much support and encouragement from the midwife and everyone around them to stay stopped, but the short- and long-term effects (Table 12.1) of quitting can sustain them.

Activity – 2

Think about a regular daily activity that gives you great pleasure and you cannot imagine your life without it, e.g.

Exercising in the gym   OR   Eating chocolate

You are told you must stop it because:

Your knee, damaged in an accident,   OR   You are diagnosed as having
has degenerated and gym work is   diabetes
making it worse

- How do you feel when the health-care professional (HCP) is really empathetic and supportive, providing you with realistic suggestions about how to manage this change?
- How do you feel when the HCP tells you that you are silly not to stop and tells you off for raising obstacles to changing your lifestyle?

TABLE 12.1 *Changes once smoking stops*

Time	Change
20 minutes	Blood pressure and pulse rate return to normal
	Circulation improves and hands and feet feel warmer
8 hours	Oxygen levels in blood return to normal
	Chances of a heart attack begin to fall
24 hours	Carbon monoxide is eliminated from the body
	Lungs start to clear mucus and other debris
48 hours	Nicotine no longer detectable in body
	Taste and smell improve
72 hours	Breathing becomes easier as bronchial tubes relax
	Energy levels increase
2–12 weeks	Circulation improves throughout the body
	Walking is easier
3–9 months	Breathing problems – cough, shortness of breath and wheezing improve
	Lung function increased by 5–10%
5 years	Risk of heart attack falls to about half of that of a smoker
10 years	Risk of lung cancer falls to about half of that of a smoker
	Risk of heart attack is about the same as someone who has never smoked

Data from Percival et al. (2003).

STRATEGIES FOR SMOKING CESSATION

How can midwives help women and their families quit smoking? The use of models of behaviour can provide a framework to guide our actions. Most simple is the 4 As (Raw et al. 1998):

- ASK the woman about smoking and her smoking habits
- ADVISE her to stop smoking

- ASSIST her by offering information and strategies
- ARRANGE referral to smoking cessation services and midwife follow-up.

These four stages can be equated to the Prochaska and DiClemente (1984) trans-theoretical stages of change model, which was developed specifically to assist professionals to support individuals with smoking cessation:

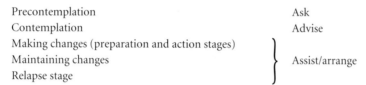

Precontemplation	Ask
Contemplation	Advise
Making changes (preparation and action stages)	
Maintaining changes	Assist/arrange
Relapse stage	

Precontemplation

Here the smoker is unaware of problems or has no interest in changing behaviour, so the midwife needs to raise awareness and perception of risks and potential problems.

Contemplation

The smoker appreciates that there is a problem, but has not decided to quit, does not want to limit her pleasure or fears failure. Midwives can help her appreciate some issues around these and why it is good to quit:

- Weigh up the benefits and costs of stopping
- Challenge misinformation
- Discuss worries about giving up
- Discuss methods of support
- Establish existing harm of smoking
- Discuss the function of smoking
- Illustrate with leaflets and information.

Having adopted a positive frame of mind and established a good rapport, to share information about the effects of smoking and benefits of stopping with the woman and her partner, the midwife uses knowledge and skills to spend quality time, perhaps for the first occasion, to address these health promotion issues. Raising the issues may be all that is possible at a first encounter to avoid information overload, but written or pictorial information can reinforce and supplement verbal interaction; supplies of leaflets and posters can be obtained from the Tobacco Information Campaign. The midwife will use her interpersonal skills to determine the best approach to take at each succeeding interaction to get the messages across.

Making changes – preparation

A single interaction with a pregnant woman is of little value without providing strategies for smoking cessation; involving her partner dramatically improves the quit rate, although HCPs are sometimes ambivalent about addressing smoking issues (Royal College of Midwives (RCM) 2002).

To help prepare the woman it is worth spending time helping her understand why she smokes; this can be achieved by the following:

- Make a smoking diary with the when and why a cigarette is smoked
- Identify high-risk times and strategies to minimize them, e.g. distractions, change of habits such as drinking juice not coffee

- Explore worries about giving up
- Write down personal goals
- Make an action plan for stopping, with specific achievable targets
- Make part of the home non-smoking
- Explore the use of NRT
- Identify treats and rewards
- Set a quit date
- Tell friends and family
- Talk to a mum who has recently stopped smoking.

These can be supported by attractive literature and leaflets.

Making changes – action

- Throw out cigarette, lighters and ashtrays
- Identify treats and rewards
- Recognize short-term benefits of having stopped (see Table 12.1)
- Have helplines and websites to hand
- NHS Pregnancy Smoking Helpline: 0800 169 9169 from 09:00 to 21:00
- NHS Smoking Helpline for partners or friends: 0800 169 0169 from 07:00 to 23:00
- NHS Direct www.nhsdirect.nhs.uk or telephone 0845 4647, 24-hour service
- Obtain NRT (bupropion is not recommended in pregnancy)
- Use usual midwife as well as specialist smoking cessation midwife, local support group or counsellor.

Withdrawal symptoms such as craving, moodiness and irritability, fidgeting, feeling lightheaded, inability to concentrate, weight gain, constipation and coughing can be explained and minimized by NRT; drinking water half-hourly, snacking on fruit and vegetables not sweets, avoiding large meals, and keeping hands and mind busy will help; coughing is a reassuring sign that the respiratory system is reactivating its defences.

Maintaining change

Continued support is vital here; motivation may be sufficient to get started, but for some staying stopped is a real challenge:

- Continued support and positive regard
- Bolster self-esteem
- Use of treats and rewards
- Carbon monoxide monitoring for visible benefits
- Identify medium-term benefits (see Table 12.1)
- Use credit card-sized reminders about the benefits
- Arrange text messages of support from friends
- Make at least four appointments for weekly face-to-face support in a group, alone or by phone
- Reinforce reasons for stopping, i.e. benefits to her and her family, how to spend the money saved
- Manage cravings with the four Ds: **d**elay, **d**eep breathe, **d**rink water, **d**o something else, read a magazine, exercise.

Government statistics use a 4-week cut-off for cessation; for pregnant women one hopes that cessation will be permanent in view of the long-term effects on the family, so ideally a follow-up at 12 months from quit date would be good to see if she is still not smoking.

Relapse

Regrettably a number of quitters will not succeed, but each time smokers stop, they are a step nearer quitting for life. It takes most smokers several attempts to succeed. The midwife should be positive about how long the woman has succeeded in stopping, even if only a few hours or days, help her by reiterating the positive benefits of stopping, and review the triggers that caused the relapse to help prepare for the next attempt when the cycle begins again.

Unfortunately many women, successful in pregnancy, relapse in the early postnatal period, but with continued midwifery support and reminders of why she stopped smoking, and reassurance that relapse is common, her self-esteem may be revitalized. Few smokers succeed in quitting at the first attempt, but the benefits to the mother and her new baby are considerable. Repeat NRT prescriptions are normally delayed for 6 months (NICE 2002) to enable time to determine the cause of the relapse, motivation to return and preparation for the next quit date to be established. Women and their partners should not be made to feel guilty or failures at relapsing, but encouraged that they succeeded for a time and that with each attempt success is more likely (RCM 2002).

Case study – 1

The journey to be a non-smoker

Shelley vividly recalls trying her first cigarette behind a tree in a park; she didn't like the taste much, but it felt exciting and wicked to a 14 year old. By 18, like her parents, she smoked regularly, she had a 10–15 a day habit; she knew it was unhealthy, but enjoyed it. In her mid-20s, an opportunistic peak flow reading indicated that Shelley retained good lung function; the HCP encouraged her to quit before it deteriorated. Shelley did and was very pleased with herself. After a year Shelley decided she could have the occasional cigarette; a few weeks later she bought a packet of 10 cigarettes to reimburse her friends and the following week it was a packet of 20 – she was hooked again. Four years later she stopped for 9 months; her relapse followed a similar pattern compounded, she claims, by stress. Eventually, aged 34, with the support of her partner and work colleagues, Shelley managed to stop for a third time; her motivation was to have a baby. She had acknowledged that she was a tobacco addict so she would never be able to smoke another cigarette without relapsing. Ten years later she remains a non-smoking mother of two healthy children.

Motivational triggers are individual and may sustain women permanently; for others motivation will be short-lived. Once the motivation to stop is identified, strategies can be suggested to realize the goal to quit smoking. The midwife can start these strategies by referring the client to a smoking cessation service or invoked if the midwife is the main HCP involved with the woman in her quest to quit (NICE 2002, West et al. 2000, RCM 2002). Identifying individual strategies for each woman and her family, providing support based on sound knowledge, with good interpersonal skills and encouragement, the midwife can help to achieve the targets set by Government and contribute positively to health promotion for the nation.

SUMMARY OF KEY POINTS

- Smoking in pregnancy is dangerous for the mother, baby and those around her.
- The midwife has a major health promotion role in identifying pregnant women who smoke and harnessing their eagerness to quit once given all the facts.
- Best results are found when advice and support are provided by specially trained smoking cessation midwives, with or without NRT.
- Quitting is difficult and all midwives need to be informed, empathetic and supportive in giving encouragement to women and their partners who wish to quit.
- Each attempt to quit brings the day of complete smoking cessation nearer, so relapse should be viewed as a step on the path to success.

REFERENCES

ASH (2004) Media briefing, Friday 12 November. Smoking and the Public Health White Paper – A license to kill? www.ash.org.uk/html/publicplaces/html/smokefreepubs.html (accessed November 2004).

Department of Health (2000) *Smoking: The facts.* London: DoH.

Department of Health (2002) *Priorities and Planning Framework 2003–2006: Improvement, expansion and reform.* London: DoH. Cited in West et al. (2003a).

Department of Health (2004a) *Summary of Intelligence on Tobacco:* www.dh.gov.uk/PublicationsAndStatistics/Publications/PublicationspolicyAndGuidance (accessed February 2005).

Department of Health (2004b) *Maternity Standard, National Service Framework for Children, Young People and Maternity Services.* London: DoH.

Department of Health (2004c) *Public Service Agreement:* www.dh.gov.uk/PublicationsAndStatistics/Publications/PublicationspolicyAndGuidance (accessed March 2005)

Department of Health (2004d) *Choosing Health: Making healthy choices easier.* London: DoH.

FOREST (2004) Briefing, Friday 12 November 2004: www.forestonline.org (accessed November 2004).

Goddard E, Higgins V (2000) *Drug Use, Smoking and Drugs Among Young Teenagers in 1999.* London: Office of National Statistics.

Hawkes, S (2004) Who is really dying for a smoke? BBC News – http//new.bbc/co/uk/go/pr/fr/-/1/hi/health/4006911.stm (accessed November 2004).

Hegaard HN, Kjærgaard H, Møller LF et al. (2004) Long-term nicotine replacement therapy. *British Journal of Midwifery* **12**: 214–20.

Markham WA, Aveyard P, Thomas H et al. (2004) What determines future smoking intentions of 12- to 13-year-old UK African-Caribbean, Indian, Pakistani and white young people. *Health Education Research Theory and Practice* **19**: 15–28.

National Institute for Clinical Excellence (2002) Guidance on the use of nicotine replacement therapy (NRT) and bupropion for smoking cessation. *Technological Appraisal Guidance No. 38.* London: NICE.

Percival J, Milner D, Wallace-Bell MA (2003) *Tobacco Control and Smoking Cessation: The role of the nurse.* Geneva: International Council of Nurses, Monograph. Cited by Wallace-Bell (2003).

Plowright N (2004) What a drag. Life health. *Observer Magazine* 7 March: 63–5.

Prochaska JO, DiClemente CC (1984) *Transtheoretical Approach: Crossing traditional boundaries of therapy.* Homewood, IL: Dow Jones/Irwin.

Raw M, McNeill A, West R (1998) Smoking cessation guidelines for health professionals. *Thorax* **53**(suppl 5, part 1): S1–19.

Rew K (2004) Constant craving. Real Life. *Observer Magazine* 17 October: 22–9.

Roberts M (2004) Passive smoking cost me dearly. Story from BBC News http://news.bbc.co.uk/go/pr/fr/-/1/hi/health/3986973.stm (accessed November 2004).

Royal College of Midwives (2002) *Helping Women Stop Smoking: A guide for midwives.* London: RCM.

Thompson KA, Parahoo KP, McCurry N et al. (2004) Women's perceptions of support from partners, family members and close friends for smoking cessation during pregnancy – combining quantitative and qualitative findings. *Health Education Research Theory and Practice* **19**: 29–39.

Twigg L, Moon G, Walker S (2004) *The Smoking Epidemic in England.* London: HDA: www.hda-online.org.uk/html/improving/smoking_epidemic.html

Wallace-Bell M (2003) Smoking cessation: the case for hospital based interventions. *Professional Nurse* **19**: 145–8.

West R, McNeill A, Raw M (2000) Smoking cessation guidelines for health professionals: an update. *Thorax* **55**: 987–99.

West R, McNeill A, Raw M (2003a) *Meeting Department of Health Smoking Cessation Targets. Recommendations for primary care trusts:* London, HDA: www.hda-online.org.uk/Documents/smoking_cessation_targets_part1.pdf (accessed February 2005).

West R, McNeill A, Raw M (2003b) *Meeting Department of Health Smoking Cessation Targets. Recommendations for service providers.* London: HAD: www.hda-online.org.uk/Documents/smoking_cessation_targets_part2.pdf

Wetter DW, Cofta-Gunn D, Irvin JE et al. (2005) What accounts for the association of education and smoking cessation? *Preventive Medicine* **40**: 452–60.

Wiseman S (2004) Stub it out. *RCN Magazine* Autumn: 12–13.

USEFUL INFORMATION AND CONTACTS

http://news.bbc.co.uk/

www.airinitiative.com

www.ash.org.uk (Action on Smoking and Health)

www.bma.org.uk/ap.nsf/content/smokefreeworld

www.forestonline.org

www.givingupsmoking.co.uk

www.dh.gov.uk/PublicationsAndStatistics

www.dh.gov.uk/PolicyAndGuidanceHealthAndSocialCareTopics/ChildrenServices/fs/en

www.hda.nhs.uk

www.nhsdirect.nhs.uk 0845 4647 is a 24-hour service

www.niceorg.uk

www.nosmokingday.co.uk

www.quit.org.uk

www.srnt.org Society for Research on Nicotine and Tobacco

NHS Pregnancy Smoking Helpline 0800 169 9169 from 09:00 to 21:00 each day

NHS Smoking Helpline 0800 169 0169 from 07:00 to 23:00 each day

Tobacco Information Campaign, PO Box 102, Hayes, Middlesex UB3 1VD, Fax 020 8867 3274

Tobacco Information Campaign Team, Room 231B, Skipton House, 80 London Road, London SE1 6LH, tel 020 7972 5313

FURTHER READING

Department of Health (1999) *Smoking Kills: A White Paper on tobacco*. London: The Stationery Office.

Department of Health (2000) *National Service Framework for Coronary Heart Disease*. London: The Stationery Office.

Department of Health (2000) *The NHS Plan. Command Paper 4818-1*. London: The Stationery Office.

Department of Health (2000) *The NHS Cancer Plan A plan for investment*. London: The Stationery Office.

Department of Health (2001) *NHS Smoking Cessation Services: Services and monitoring guidance 2001/2*. London: DoH.

Department of Health (2001) *Statistics on Smoking Cessation Services in Health Authorities: England, April 2000–March 2001*. London: Government Statistical Service.

Department of Health (2002) *Priorities and Planning Framework 2003–2006: Improvement, expansion and reform*. London: DoH.

Department of Health (2002) *Service and Monitoring Guidance Note 2001/2–2002: Shifting the balance: Reforms and monitoring for 2002/03*. London: DoH.

Gleeson C, Memon I, Milner M, Baines S (1997) Smoking cessation in pregnancy: a multiple contact approach. *British Journal of Midwifery* **5**: 551–4.

Health Development Agency (2003) *Standard for Training in Smoking Cessation Treatments*. London: HDA.

Pullon S, McLeod D, Benn C et al. (2003) Smoking cessation in New Zealand: education and resources for use by midwives for women who smoke during pregnancy. *Health Promotion International* **18**: 315–25.

Woods SE, Lake JR, Springett J (2003) Tackling health inequalities and the HAZ Smoking Cessation Programme: the perfect match? *Critical Public Health* **13**: 61–76.

13 THE CHALLENGE OF MENTAL HEALTH PROMOTION

JAN BOWDEN AND VICKY MANNING

Mental health and mental ill-health have become a central aspect of care within midwifery in recent years, especially with the recent data from the sixth report Why Mothers Die *(Lewis and Drife 2004) indicating that mental ill-health is now the leading cause of death in a pregnant or postpartum woman. Midwives, as the lead professionals for most of the care provided by maternity services in the UK, need to have a greater awareness of mental health and its impact on a woman's health, which extends beyond just knowledge of the 'baby blues', postnatal depression and puerperal psychosis. They need to develop skills in mental health promotion as well as skills to assess and refer women accordingly. However, mental health, and in particular mental ill-health, suffers from prejudicial and stigmatizing attitudes (Crisp et al. 2000, Royal College of Psychiatrists (RCOP) 2000). Add to that the taboo nature of maternal suicides and the need to move emotional care beyond a superficial level and difficulties arise. Midwives, similar to everyone else, have their own personal constructs, attitudes, and ethical and moral judgements about mental health, which can and will impact on this area of care. This chapter explores these issues and examines the effects that mental health loss has on the relationship of the woman and her partner and their baby, and identifies the role of the midwife in mental health promotion, screening for mental ill-health and supporting women when they become mentally unwell.*

THE BACKGROUND TO MENTAL HEALTH AND MIDWIFERY

The most recent *Why Mothers Die* report (Lewis and Drife 2004) has again highlighted the real impact of mental illness and suicide on the maternal death rates. Worrying new data have indicated that more women than before are committing

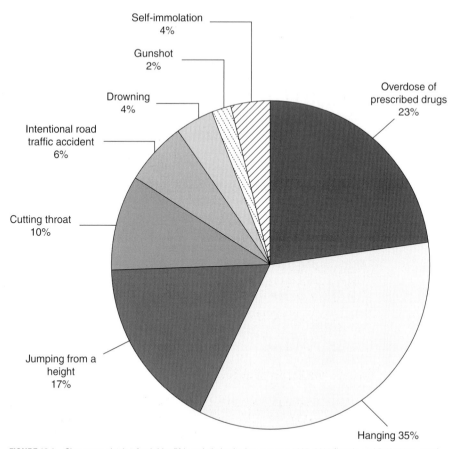

FIGURE 13.1 *Chosen methods of suicide: fifth and sixth trinnium reports 1997–2002 (Lewis and Drife 2001, 2004)*

suicide. Alarm bells are also ringing in regard to the ways in which the suicides are being carried out – they are very violent – and a violent suicide has always been considered to be traditionally a male trait (Hawton 2000). It had always been considered that a newborn infant and/or her other children would act as a deterrent and prevent a mother from committing suicide. Evidence now shows that this assumption may no longer be the case (Appleby 1991, RCOP 2000).

In the previous report, a rise in suicides in the years 1997–99 from 1/100 000 maternities to 2/100 000 maternities was noted (Lewis and Drife 2001). The report recorded that there were 42 deaths as a result of mental illness, which included 27 suicides. The current report (Lewis and Drife 2004) has identified a further increase in the number of deaths caused by mental illness from 42 to 60 deaths, which include 26 suicides, most of which were violent (Figure 13.1). The fifth and sixth reports highlighted the following recommendations (Lewis and Drife 2001, 2004):

- All women booking their pregnancy should be asked detailed questions about their current mental health and mental health history, including self-harm, domestic violence, eating disorders, drug and alcohol misuse, and family history of mental illness.
- A psychiatrist should assess all women with a previous mental health history in the antenatal period and a plan of care instigated.

- A perinatal mental health team that has specialist knowledge, skills and experience in dealing with women at risk of or suffering from serious mental illness post partum should be available to every woman.
- Women who have had a mental illness either after childbirth or at any other time in their lives should be counselled as to the possible risk of a recurrence.
- Women who require admission for psychiatric treatment should ideally be admitted to a specialized mother and baby unit together with their infants. If this is unavailable transfer to the nearest available unit must be considered.
- Substance misuse services, without the need for an appointment, should be provided in the antenatal clinic. This will assist with increasing the rate of client engagement with the service and compliance with care.
- The term 'postnatal depression' (PND) should not be used as a generic term for all types of mental illness.
- Future enquiries must require the collection of information from mental health services in cases where mental illness is a cause of maternal death.
- There is a need for perinatal psychiatry to be included in the professional development of midwives, obstetricians and general practitioners (GP).
- Training should be put into place before routine screening of serious mental illness is instigated.
- Midwives, obstetricians and GPs should have an awareness of the laws and issues pertaining to child protection.

Chosen methods of suicide

Current evidence shows that between 15 and 25 per cent of childbearing women are likely to develop a clinically consequential mental health disorder in the interval between conception and the end of the first year of being a mother (Priest et al. 2005). Perinatal disorders include minor and major depressions, anxiety disorders and panic attacks (Glover and O'Connor 2002), post-traumatic stress disorder (Callahan and Hynan 2002), bipolar disorder and schizophrenia (Oates 2003). These mental health problems are often entangled with the complexities of drug/alcohol abuse and domestic violence (Carter et al. 2003, Doggett et al. 2003, Bacchus et al. 2004). These issues can cause intense distress to the woman, her partner and her family, and can have long-lasting effects on the woman, on her partner and on the cognitive, emotional and behavioural development of the child, with an increased risk of suicide (Murray and Cooper 1997, Murray and Hamilton 2005).

DEFINING MENTAL HEALTH AND MENTAL HEALTH PROMOTION

Activity – 1

- Consider your definitions of mental health and mental health promotion.
- Write them down before reading this section.
- Identify what influenced your definitions.
- Do you feel that you work with these definitions in your current role?

Health is affected when the potent balance of an individual's make-up is unable to make adaptations to a frequently changing internal and external environment. This balance is particularly delicate in the area of mental health and nowhere is it so far reaching in the effects of its breakdown. Any upsets in the mental health of a woman around the time of childbirth will affect not only the woman, but also her partner, her family, including her child, and her whole social setting.

As identified in Chapter 3, how to define and interpret health has been a subject of debate and impasse for a significant period of time (Illich 1975, World Health Organization (WHO) 1984, 1985). Mental health is even more difficult to define. A wide scope of emotional and behavioural reactions can be seen in people responding to similar events or circumstances. Cultural factors and the social context in which mental health is understood will further complicate these responses and their meaning (Adams 1997).

Definitions of mental health vary and have incorporated the potential to grow and develop, lead a settled life, and identify the need for inner psychological health and the ability to approach problems in a way that is acceptable to tradition and society while holding on to a rational viewpoint (Caplan 1961, Maslow 1968, Neumann et al. 1989). This reveals the subjective nature of the concept of mental health and the difficulty in trying to develop a stand-alone definition.

Other authors have gone along the path of choosing to define mental health by highlighting a criteria-driven definition that includes: coping skills to adapt to life changes; the ability to identify stressors and effect a constructive response; the development of the concept of 'self'; the impact of self-esteem and worthiness; and the degree of social support (Tudor 1996, Telford et al. 1997). These criteria-driven definitions have their own problems in that it is not always clear how many of these criteria an individual has to have to be judged either mentally well or mentally ill.

Other authors have argued that a definition of mental health has to include biological issues and genetic predispositions, gender and ethnicity issues, socioeconomic and environmental issues, and family dynamics (Soni Raleigh et al. 1990, WHO 1992, Tudor 1996, Department of Health (DoH) 1998).

It may be easier, in practical terms, to look at the opposite of mental health and define mental illness instead. From the evidence, this appears to be the easiest option and one of the simplest definitions of mental illness is by Kendall and Zealley (1993), who define it as the disorder of memory, perception, cognition, mood and will.

Given the lack of unity regarding the definition of mental health and what constitutes mental health, we have come to the challenge of how to define mental health promotion. In Chapter 3 the concept of health promotion has been explored and, as with health, health promotion and its definition can at times appear to lack a consensus. It is concerned with the activities that improve the health status of the individual, the community and the population at large, including the activities of health education, environmental and social change, empowerment and advocacy.

Hodgson et al. (1996) embraced the viewpoint that mental health promotion is the application of interventions that could be applied to the population as a whole. This approach would appear to fit the requirements of midwives whose role it is to promote the mental health of all their clients, and especially to those at risk of developing or who currently have a mental health problem.

Perhaps the difficulty in finding a suitable and workable definition of mental health and mental health promotion is tied into the multiple factors that contribute to mental health, how mental illness is viewed and the way in which these views often lead to stigma and collusion. The next sections look at the factors affecting mental health attitudes and mental health.

FACTORS AFFECTING MENTAL HEALTH

Activity – 2

- List the factors that you feel may affect a woman's mental health in a positive way.
- List the factors that you feel may affect a woman's mental health in a negative way (see Box 13.2 for the authors' suggestions).

Similar to physical health, mental health is affected by a multitude of factors that can impact upon an individual in a positive or a negative way. How that individual copes with these factors often depends on what is happening in her life at the time, her life experiences, and her ability to instigate and cope with change. Add to this the maelstrom of pregnancy, childbirth and becoming a parent, and the impact to a woman's mental health is hugely significant. Midwives need to be proactive, anticipating aspects that may adversely affect a woman's mental health so that early support can be offered. This includes risk assessment and being aware of the most vulnerable groups (Box 13.1), so care can be targeted and early support offered (DoH 2001, 2002).

VULNERABLE GROUPS

Research into these factors has led to apparently conflicting views, because objectively measuring emotions, attitudes and behaviour is difficult. Contributing causes have, however, emerged under the main categories of psychosocial factors, biological factors, psychiatric/emotional factors, obstetric/gynaecological factors and infant factors (Priest et al. 2005).

Box 13.1 Groups identified as vulnerable and needing specific mental health provision

Particularly vulnerable groups	Groups requiring specific mental health provision
Mothers and carers	Dual diagnosis of substance misuse
Older women	Perinatal mental ill-health
Black and ethnic minority women	Eating disorders
Lesbian and bisexual women	Women offenders
Transsexual women	Experience of violence and abuse
Women involved in prostitution	Self-harm
Women offenders	Diagnosis of borderline personality disorder
Women with learning disabilities	
Women with alcohol and drug misuse	

Adapted from *Women's Mental Health into the Mainstream* (DoH 2002)

Psychosocial factors

Psychosocial factors include life stressors such as bereavement, separation/lone parent, unemployment, illness, moving house, lack of social support and domestic violence (Riley 1995, Bacchus et al. 2004, Priest et al. 2005).

Relationship factors

A poor relationship with husband/partner or marital instability is considered a risk factor for loss of mental health for mothers (Levy and Kline 1994, Schaper et al. 1994, Priest et al. 2005).

Social support

A large longitudinal study by Williams et al. (1981) in the general field of mental health came to these conclusions:

- Effective social support systems predict improvements in mental health over a period of time.
- Negative life events and physical limitations predict a deterioration in mental health over time.

There is a requirement in the booking interview that midwives try to discover the social support available to women, particularly those in the vulnerable groups. The weaker the support network, the more likely the woman is to report illness (physical and emotional) both during her pregnancy and postnatally. Social capital influences aspects of mental health and its promotion as it does physical health (Putnam 1993, 1995, DoH 2001).

Relationship with own mother

Raphael-Leff (1991) considers that this relationship is of central importance in maternalization. She reports sadness and feelings of deprivation where a woman has lost her own mother during childhood from death, divorce or separation. Some of her observations of new mothers showed that they did not have as much interaction with their babies as women who still had a mother. The lack of a role model can also affect their behaviour towards the babies. Murray et al. (1995) found that postnatal depression was more likely to occur in women who had a poor relationship with their mothers, whereas in other forms of depression within a control group there was no such definite association.

Biological factors

There is very little evidence that there is a biological basis for mental ill-health during childbearing (Cooper and Murray 1998). Mood changes can occur with both hypo- and hyperthyroidism and, according to Riley (1995), 20 per cent of postnatal women have mild dysfunction of the thyroid. Most commonly a degree of hyperthyroidism occurs between 1 and 4 months after delivery and hypothyroidism after the fourth month. A small number of such women will suffer from PND.

Psychiatric/emotional factors

Pregnancy is a time of change, psychological and physical. It is normal for women to experience a wide gamete of emotions such as anxiety over the changes in her life or whether she will be a good mother (Cantwell and Cox 2003). Women who have experienced postnatal depression in previous pregnancies are at an increased risk of experiencing it again (Cooper and Murray 1995), although the evidence does not define the risk clearly, presenting it at 25–75 per cent (Watson et al. 1984). There is stronger evidence that 'the blues' are related to PND. Many of the women who experience severe baby blues go on to develop PND (O'Hara 1997).

A qualitative study by Green (1990) that looked at mood rather than depression found that women who were happy to be pregnant remained happy in the puerperium. Unhappiness was increased by feelings of lack of control in labour, lack of involvement in decision-making and that interventions were not right for them.

Obstetric/gynaecological factors

Some research has been carried out to investigate the connection between various obstetric and gynaecological factors and mental ill-health. The evidence for making the link between traumatic/difficult delivery and PND is limited. Generally, obstetric interventions, such as induction or forceps delivery, do not appear to carry a risk unless, as already mentioned, the woman did not feel them to be right for her (Green 1990). Menage (1996) studied 500 women, of whom one-fifth had had a distressing obstetric or gynaecological procedure. She considered 1.5 per cent could be diagnosed as suffering from post-traumatic stress disorder (PTSD). Another small study of 171 women suggests that the women who perceive the pain of labour as extreme are more at risk of PND (Goldstein Ferber et al. 2005). The health of the baby may also affect the mental health of the mother with depression associated with neonatal risk, stillbirth, neonatal death or sudden infant death and very-low birthweight (Bennett and Slade 1991, Boyle et al. 1996, O'Brian et al. 1999, Singer et al. 1999).

FACTORS THAT MAY AFFECT MATERNAL MENTAL HEALTH

Compare the list in Box 13.2 with your list. Our list is far from definitive and you may have different items. What needs to be remembered is that women who may be

---

Box 13.2   Factors that may affect maternal mental health

Positive	Negative
High education achievement	Low education achievement
Employment	Unemployed
Having a home	Stressed at work
Having a supportive partner	Homeless
Planned pregnancy	Living in a 'poor' area
Good relationship with own mother	Poor social support
Live in a 'nice' area	Poor relationship with mother
Child care facilities	Domestic violence
Giving up work	Unsupportive partner
	Unplanned pregnancy
	Fertility problems before conception
	Having two or more children
	Giving up work
	Recent bereavement(s)
	Previous mental health issues

seen as 'having it all' may become depressed, and those who have many negative factors in their lives may not. Anyone felt to be at risk should be referred with her consent to specialists for support.

ATTITUDES AND MENTAL HEALTH

The midwife's attitudes

All human beings develop attitudes; this process starts as children, and is influenced by many factors such as parents, peers, schoolteachers and the media. These attitudes may develop into prejudice, which may affect how a midwife may react when first meeting a woman whose culture, ethnicity, class, habits or social functioning differs from her own 'normal'.

Midwives need to be aware of their own prejudices so that they can practise with an open, non-judgemental, un-biased approach. This will help to ensure that each woman feels able to disclose very personal information where this is appropriate. However, this is not as simple as it appears and, where a prejudice arises, it is important to develop a strategy to cope with it and allow the adoption of an open and unbiased approach, or to know about referring to colleagues when this is not possible and there is a risk that a client's care will be affected.

Limited research indicates that, similar to other health-care professionals, midwives like looking after certain types of clients. The most liked were women who were clean, cheerful, open-minded, cooperative, ordinary and good communicators and those who were appreciative! The most commonly disliked women were those perceived as dirty or smelly, professionals such as teachers and lawyers, those who were rude and aggressive, those with no sense of humour or seen as inflexible, and those who failed to recognize the status of the midwife. Those who were disadvantaged or with mental health problems did not appear to raise strong feelings either way (Roberts 1984).

However, mental health and mental ill-health have for many years suffered with the tags of stigmatization, prejudice and collusion within society and, as the midwife is from that society, her understanding of mental health may be flavoured by societal views, as well as her own community and personal experiences of mental health (O'Hara and Swain 1996, Crisp et al. 2000, RCOP 2000).

THE EFFECTS OF MENTAL HEALTH LOSS

Antenatal mental ill-health

Recent work has looked at the emotional and psychological factors during pregnancy, which may affect the relationship that a woman has with her child. Findings appear to show that there is a correlation between the woman's ability to bond with her baby and her psychological and emotional well-being during the antenatal period. Mental health issues can have physical and emotional consequences for mother and infant (Spietz and Kelly 2002):

- Domestic violence can result in low birthweight.
- Maternal depression has been linked to depression-like symptoms in newborns.
- Pre-term labour can often be attributed to psychosomatic or psychosocial issues such as stress.
- Some stress hormones are thought to interfere with fetal brain development.

On mother–infant interaction

There are many reasons for delayed attachment to a baby in those mothers who appear to be in a 'normal' state of mental health. Such reasons include the separation of the mother and baby immediately after birth, the 'wrong' sex or a baby with an untoward appearance, particularly when some facial abnormality is apparent. Babies vary in both appearance and behaviour, with some babies, for instance, being more 'cuddly' than others. Newborn babies show rapid adaptation and have the capacity actively to seek and regulate a response from the closest consistent caretaker, usually the mother. There is increasing evidence that poor postnatal maternal mental health not only affects the woman, but can also affect the child.

Current research clearly shows an association connecting to the health and development of the child. Maternal mental illness can have a major impact on maternal child bonding (Atkinson and Zucker 1997): the cognitive, emotional, social and behavioural development of the child (Barnett et al. 1993, Murray and Cooper 1997, Cooper and Murray 1998, Huizuik et al. 2002, McLennan and Offord 2002, O'Connor et al. 2002, Carter et al. 2003). This particularly appears to affect male children, who may continue to have emotional and behavioural problems well into their late teens (Glover and O'Connor 2002). Women who are non-English speaking also become depressed and one small study has shown that they are not supported as well as English-speaking women. The affects on their children can then be compounded by the difficulty that health professionals may have in assessing development. The use of interpreters is essential to ensure that services are provided to their full capacity (Foss et al. 2004).

The birth of a new baby is a critical, sensitive time for all family members. Both parents are trying to adapt to their lifestyle changes and relationship. The woman's income may reduce or disappear and this may create an adverse financial situation. This may cause the father stress, compounded because his home responsibilities may increase (Riley 1995). Ballard et al. (1994) reported that 9 per cent of fathers were found to be depressed 6 weeks after a new baby's birth and 5.4 per cent by 6 months. This in turn may delay the mother's recovery and affect the child or children's development (Murray et al. 1991). It is possible that some men may need counselling or treatment to enable them to support the family. Researchers, health-care professionals and the media had largely overlooked the effect on the father of PND, and indeed his own risk of developing depression after the birth of a child.

THE ROLE OF THE MIDWIFE

Mental health promotion, screening for mental illness and supporting women with mental health issues

Mental health is a difficult area to promote and this, as we have seen, is partly the result of the attitudes that accompany mental health of health professionals and the lay population alike, and the development of stigma, prejudice and collusion. The midwife is in an ideal position to break down the barriers that surround mental health and to promote and normalize it. The role would be applicable to all the midwife's clients and especially for those at risk of developing mental health issues and those currently with mental health issues. Mental health promotion falls into three areas.

Primary mental health promotion

Primary mental health promotion is concerned with the promotion and normalization of mental health and the breaking down of negative barriers surrounding mental health in the general healthy population. It looks at ways in which the positive and negative influences on mental health can be identified and pinpoint ways in which these influences can be encouraged or discouraged.

Mental illness can be explored, allowing myths surrounding mental illness to be dispelled and to identify where help and support can be sought. It also involves the promotion of the ability of individuals to look after and maintain their own mental health (Keeley 2002). Examples of this in midwifery practice would be talking about the 'blues' and PND in an antenatal education class, having up-to-date literature readily available for women to pick up and read, and workshops or study days for the midwives to attend to start the normalization and promotion of the mental health process.

Secondary mental health promotion

Secondary mental health promotion is concerned with the early detection of mental illness in those vulnerable groups of people who are at risk of developing mental health issues. Part of this promotion will be to normalize and break down barriers that affect mental health, but this time targeted at a specific group of women rather than at the population as a whole (Keeley 2002). This will hopefully aid the prevention of stigma and collusion that are a major problem within mental health and midwifery (O'Hara and Swain 1996, RCOP 2000, Lewis and Drife 2001). An example of this in midwifery practice would be the assessment of mental health during the antenatal period and referral to the psychiatric/mental health team. This is now a recommendation of the *Why Women Die* report (Lewis and Drife 2001, 2004) and should have been implemented across maternity services in the UK. However, there are several issues that need to be explored.

First, what mental health assessment tool should be used? All booking interview templates should now contain questions pertaining to mental illness with supplementary questions about whether the illness was inside or outside of pregnancy, length of illness, treatment, whether admitted for treatment and at what unit, and recurrences if any. There is current debate about whether the Edinburgh Post Natal Depression Scale (EPNDS) should be used in both antenatal and postnatal periods by midwives. It would be used to provide a baseline assessment of the woman's feelings and moods for the health visitors who undertake the late postnatal EPNDS, when PND is more likely. There are some, however, who feel that the current use of the EPNDS is unable to pick up the amount of PND that it was hoped to as a result of its limited success in ethnic minority groups (Seeley 2001). It would normalize mental health because it would target the whole pregnant population as well as identifying clearly to the woman that issues surrounding mental health can be discussed with her midwife without judgement being made. It would also provide a tool to identify antenatal depression, which has recently been identified within the research as an area of perinatal psychiatry that has been neglected (Seeley 2001, Coyle and Adams 2002), although it has been identified that this is not the intended use of the EPNDS.

Second, there is the question of training for the midwives who will be expected to provide this service. Provision of knowledge will not be enough; attitudes and behaviour need to be addressed. Midwives need to reflect on their practice, attitudes and knowledge, and focus on how they can deal with the needs of women (and themselves) where there is heightened emotional care (Murray and Hamilton 2005). Psychological care requires a much deeper level of therapeutic commitment. It needs time for the woman to tell her story, it requires good assessment and referral skills on the part of the midwife, and it necessitates good pathways of care to be in place to support those in whom a mental health issue has been identified (DoH 2001, 2002).

The Maternal and Perinatal Partnerships in Mental Health (MAPPIM) project has started to address these concerns. This project serves an area that is culturally diverse and has many socioeconomic disadvantages that are known to affect mental health. The MAPPIM project's overall aim is to provide a seamless mental health service for all women booking for care at Guy's and St Thomas' Hospitals. A mental health assessment on all pregnant women at booking is undertaken. Discovery of a mental health issue is addressed by the development of a well-coordinated multi-agency care pathway. It also ensures perinatal mental health assessment and management, continuity of care, and a 24-hour response to acute episodes for mentally unwell women that is specialist consultant led. Under the project, all the midwives will be trained to detect and manage mental health, as well as substance misuse problems, thus providing the advice, support, care and treatment that these women need (Murray and Hamilton 2005). This particular aim is important considering the recommendations of the sixth report (Lewis and Drife 2004).

Tertiary mental health promotion

Tertiary mental health promotion is the final aspect of mental health promotion and is concerned with the provision of interventions and instigation of care for those who have a current or enduring mental health issue (Keeley 2002). Again part of this promotion will be to normalize and break down barriers but its key area is the early detection and referral to a specialist team to allow for assessment, treatment and the instigation of a care plan. The midwife, in this area of mental health promotion, may find herself acting as an advocate for her client, as well as using her communication skills to converse with a multidisciplinary team and working in partnership with other agencies that go beyond her normal boundaries of practice. An example of this in midwifery practice would be the midwife who works within a case loading team that specializes in those clients with a psychiatric illness (Bloom 2001).

There are many examples of good practice. Since 1989 the Brierley Midwifery Practice at King's College Hospital NHS Trust has given care to those women who have mental health problems. Continuity of care right through pregnancy, delivery and up to 28 days' postnatal help provides stability and security to those who often lack both in their lives. The practice has regular meetings with a senior psychiatric registrar and the perinatal consultant as well as the obstetrician, who is available for advice. The midwives liaise with the community psychiatric nursing teams and foster strong links with the mother and baby unit at the local psychiatric hospital to ensure continuation of midwifery care if a woman requires admission (Kumar et al. 1995, Meyer and Wallace 1995).

SUMMARY OF KEY POINTS

- The latest *Why Mothers Die* report (Lewis and Drife 2004) has revealed that mental health, and suicides in particular, remain a leading cause of maternal death.
- Mental health issues will affect the health of the women, her partner and her child.
- Mental health promotion is an urgent area that midwives need to address within their practice.
- Stigmatization, prejudice and collusion are tags that, even today, are still very much attached to mental health and mental ill-health, which leads to problems such as fear, ignorance and stereotypes.
- Midwives can be active in primary, secondary and tertiary mental health promotion, by allowing mental health to be normalized and more openly discussed within midwifery practice by midwives, women and their families without fear of a judgement call being made. It also allows those women with mental health issues to be identified early and an appropriate referral to be made. For those women who are mentally unwell, it will ensure instigation of an appropriate, agreed, multi-professional care and treatment plan.

REFERENCES

Adams M (1997) The challenges of mental health promotion. In: Crafter H (ed.), *Health Promotion in Midwifery Practice.* London: Arnold, pp. 228–61.

Appleby L (1991) Suicide during pregnancy and in the first postnatal year. *British Medical Journal* **302**: 137–40.

Atkinson L, Zucker KJ (1997) *Attachment and Psychopathology.* New York: Guilford Press.

Bacchus L, Mezey G, Bewley S (2004) Domestic violence: prevalence in pregnant women and associations with physical and psychological health. *European Journal of Obstetrics and Gynaecology and Reproductive Biology* **113**: 6–11.

Ballard C, Davis R, Dean C (1994) Study in postnatal depression in mothers and fathers. In Recent Advances in Childbearing and Mental Health. Abstracts of the Sixth International Conference of the Marcé Society. *British Journal of Psychiatry* **164**: 782–8.

Barnett B, Lockhart K, Bernard D, Maricavasagar V, Dudley M (1993) Mood disorders among infants of mothers admitted to a mother craft hospital. *Journal of Paediatrics and Child Health* **29**: 270–5.

Bennett DE, Slade P (1991) Infants born at risk: consequences for maternal post-partum adjustment. *British Journal of Medical Psychology* **64**: 159–72.

Bloom J (2001) Midwifery and perinatal mental health care provision. *British Journal of Midwifery* **9**: 385–8.

Boyle FM, Vance JC, Najman JM, Thearle MJ (1996) The mental health impact of stillbirth, neonatal death or SIDS: prevalence and patterns of distress among mothers. *Social Science and Medicine* **43**: 1273–82.

Callahan JL, Hynan MT (2002) Identifying mothers at risk for postnatal emotional distress: further evidence for the validity of the perinatal posttraumatic stress disorder questionnaire. *Journal of Perinatology* **31**: 349–57.

Cantwell R, Cox JL (2003) Psychiatric disorders in pregnancy and the puerperium. *Current Obstetrics and Gynaecology* **13**: 7–13.

Caplan G (1961) *An Approach to Community Mental Health.* London: Tavistock.

Carter AS, Garrity-Roukas FE, Chazan-Cohen R, Little C, Broggs-Gowan M (2003) Maternal depression and co-morbidity: predicting early parenting, attachment security and toddler social-emotional problems and competencies. *Journal of the American Academy of Child and Adolescence Psychiatry* **40**: 18–26.

Cooper PJ, Murray L (1995) The course and recurrence of postnatal depression. *British Journal of Psychiatry* **166**: 191–5.

Cooper PJ, Murray L (1998) Postnatal depression. *British Medical Journal* **316**: 1884–6.

Coyle B, Adams C (2002) The EPNDS: Guidelines for its use as part of a Maternal Mood Assessment. *Community Practitioner* **75**: 394–5.

Crisp AH, Gelder MG, Rix S (2000) Stigmatisation of people with mental illnesses. *British Journal of Psychiatry* **177**: 4–7.

Department of Health (1998) *Our Healthier Nation: A contract for health.* London: HMSO.

Department of Health (2001) *Making it Happen. A guide to delivering mental health promotion.* London: DoH.

Department of Health (2002) *Women's Mental Health into the Mainstream. Strategic development of mental health care for women: summary.* London: DoH.

Doggett C, Burrett S, Michaels C, Osborn DA (2003) Home visits during pregnancy and postpartum for women with an alcohol and/or drug problem. *The Cochrane Database of Systematic Reviews* 2003, Issue 3. Art No D004456.DOI:10.1002/1465185.CD004456.

Foss GF, Chantel AW, Hendrickson S (2004) Maternal depression and anxiety and infant development: A comparison of foreign-born and native-born mothers. *Public Health Nursing* **21**: 237–46.

Glover V, O'Connor TG (2002) Effects of antenatal stress and anxiety. *British Journal of Psychiatry* **180**: 389–91.

Goldstein Ferber S, Granot M, Zimmer EZ (2005) Catastrophizing labour pain compromises later maternity adjustments. *American Journal of Obstetrics and Gynecology* **192**: 826–31.

Green J (1990) Who is unhappy after childbirth? Antenatal and intrapartum correlates from a prospective study. *Journal of Reproductive and Infant Psychology* **8**: 175–83.

Hawton K (2000) Sex and suicide: gender differences in suicidal behaviour. *British Journal of Psychiatry* **177**: 484–5.

Hodgson RJ, Abbasi T, Clarkson J (1996) Effective mental health promotion: a literature review. *Health Education Journal* **55**: 55–74.

Huizuik AC, De Robles-Medina PG, Mulder EJH, Visser GHA (2002) Psychological measures of prenatal stress as predictors of infant temperament. *Journal of the American Academy of Child and Adolescent Psychiatry* **41**: 1078–85.

Illich I (1975) *Medical Nemesis.* London: Calder & Boyers.

Keeley P (2002) Mental health promotion. In: Kerr J (ed.), *Community Health Promotion Challenges for Practice.* London: Baillière Tindall, pp. 183–205.

Kendall R, Zealley A (1993) *Companion to Psychiatric Studies*, Vol 5. Edinburgh: Churchill Livingstone.

Kumar R, Marks M, Jackson K (1995) Prevention and treatment of postnatal psychiatric disorders. *British Journal of Midwifery* **3**: 314–17.

Lewis G, Drife J (eds) (2001) *Why Mothers Die 1997–1999: The Fifth Report of the Confidential Enquiries into Maternal Deaths in the United Kingdom.* London: RCOG Press.

Lewis G, Drife J (eds) (2004) *Why Mothers Die 2000–2002. The Sixth Report of the Confidential Enquiries into Maternal Deaths in the United Kingdom.* London: RCOG Press.

Levy V, Kline P (1994) Perinatal depression: a factor analysis. *British Journal of Midwifery* **2**: 154–9.

McLennan JD, Offord DR (2002) Should postpartum depression be targeted to improve child mental health. *Journal of the American Academy of Child and Adolescent Psychiatry* **41**: 28–35.

Maslow AH (1968) *Towards a Psychology of Being.* New York: Van Nostrand.

Menage J (1996) Post-traumatic stress disorder may follow childbirth. *British Medical Journal* **313**: 28.

Meyer J, Wallace V (1995) Mothers' help. *Nursing Times* **91**: 42–3.

Murray D, Cox D, Chapman G, Jones P (1995) Childbirth: life event or start of long term difficulty? Further data from the Stoke on Trent controlled study of postnatal depression. *British Journal of Psychiatry* **166**: 595–600.

Murray K, Hamilton S (2005) Perinatal mental health: a Northern Ireland perspective. *MIDIRS Midwifery Digest* **15**: 121–4.

Murray L, Cooper PJ (1997) Postpartum depression and child development. *Psychological Medicine* **27**: 253–60.

Murray L, Cooper PJ, Stein A (1991) Postnatal depression and infant development. *British Medical Journal* **309**: 378–9.

Neumann J, Schroeder H, Voss P (1989) *Mental Health and Wellbeing: The context of the health promotion concept.* Copenhagen: WHO.

Oates M (2003) Perinatal psychiatric disorders: a leading cause of maternal morbidity and mortality. *British Medical Bulletin* **67**: 219–29.

O'Brian M, Hero Asay J, McCluskey-Fawcett K (1999) Family functioning and maternal depression following premature birth. *Journal of Reproduction and Infant Psychology* **17**: 178–88.

O'Connor TG, Heron J, Golding J, Beveridge M, Glover V (2002) Maternal antenatal anxiety and children's behavioural/emotional problems at 4 years: report from the ALSPAC. *British Journal of Psychiatry* **180**: 502–8.

O'Hara MW (1997) The nature of postpartum depressive disorders. In: Murray L, Cooper PJ (eds), *Postpartum Depression and Child Development.* New York: Guilford, pp. 3–31.

O'Hara MW, Swain AM (1996) Rates and risks of post partum depression – a meta-analysis. *International Review of Psychiatry* **8**: 37–54.

Priest SR, Austin M, Sullivan E (2005) Antenatal psychosocial screening for prevention of antenatal and postnatal anxiety and depression (Protocol). *The Cochrane Collaboration.* Chichester: Wiley & Sons Ltd.

Putnam R (1993) *Bowling Alone: The collapse and revival of American community.* New York: Simon & Schuster.

Putnam R (1995) Bowling alone: America's declining social capital. *Journal of Democracy* **6**: 65–78.

Raphael-Leff J (1991) *Psychological Processes of Childbearing.* London: Chapman & Hall.

Riley D (1995) *Perinatal Mental Health: A source book for professionals.* Oxford: Radcliffe Medical Press.

Roberts D (1984) Non-verbal communication. Popular and unpopular patients. In: Faulkner A (ed.), *Communication.* Edinburgh: Churchill Livingstone, pp. 12–17.

Royal College of Psychiatrists (2000) *Perinatal Maternal Mental Health Services. Council Report CR88.* London: RCOP.

Schaper A, Rooney B, Kay N, Silva P (1994) Use of the Edinburgh postnatal depression scale to identify postpartum depression in a clinical setting. *Journal of Reproductive Medicine* **139**: 620–4.

Seeley S (2001) Strengths and limitations of the postnatal depression screening scale. In: *Post Natal Depression and Maternal Mental Health: A public health priority.* CPHVA Conference Proceedings. London: Community Practitioners' and Health Visitors' Association.

Singer LT, Salvator A, Guo S et al. (1999) Maternal psychological distress and parenting stress after the birth of a very low-birth weight infant. *JAMA* **281**: 799–805.

Soni Raleigh V, Bulusu L, Balarajan R (1990) Suicides among immigrant from the Indian sub-continent. *British Journal of Psychiatry* **156**: 46–50.

Spietz A, Kelly J (2002) The importance of maternal mental health during pregnancy: theory, practice and intervention. *Public Health Nursing* **19**: 153–5.

Telford S, Delancey F, Vogels M (1997) *Effectiveness of Mental Health Promotion Interventions: A review*. London: Health Education Authority.

Tudor K (1996) *Mental Health Promotion: Paradigms and practice*. London: Routledge.

Watson J, Elliot S, Rugg A, Brough D (1984) Psychiatric disorder in pregnancy and the first postnatal year. *British Journal of Psychiatry* **144**: 454–62.

Williams A, Ware J, Donald C (1981) A model of mental health, life events and social supports applicable to General Populations. *Journal of Health and Social Behaviour* **22**: 324–36.

World Health Organization (1984) *Health Promotion. A discussion document on the concepts and principles*. Copenhagen: WHO.

World Health Organization (1985) *Targets for Health for All*. Copenhagen: WHO.

World Health Organization (1992) *Health for All*. Copenhagen: WHO.

FURTHER READING

Department of Health (2001) *Making It Happen: A guide to delivering mental health promotion*. London: DoH.

WEBSITE

SIGN guidelines on postnatal depression and puerperal psychosis (2000): www.sign.ac.uk/guidelines/fulltext/60/section1.html

14 DOMESTIC VIOLENCE AND HEALTH PROMOTION: MIDWIVES CAN MAKE A DIFFERENCE

GILL ASTON

Research has highlighted that domestic violence is a major health problem impacting on the health status of women and the utilization rates for health and reproductive care services. Increased understanding of the relationship between domestic violence and health has resulted in national and professional strategies calling for an enhanced midwifery role in maximizing the health of women experiencing domestic violence. Midwives have been identified as often being especially well placed to be able to identify and help tackle the problem of domestic violence (Royal College of Midwives 1997, Department of Health (DoH) 2000, Price et al. 2005). During the course of their clinical practice midwives are in a unique and important position to create safe clinical environments for assessing and effectively responding to domestic violence. The nature of the relationship between a woman and her midwife, and the fact that virtually every woman is seen by a midwife not once but many times during pregnancy, labour and after childbirth, means that a strong case has been made for midwives to enquire about domestic violence in maternity care settings (Price 2003, DoH 2004, Salmon et al. 2004).

The experience of domestic violence may result in a number of women's health problems during the childbearing years. Research that has examined the impact of domestic violence on women's physical and mental health has found that women with a history of domestic violence are more likely to experience a wide range of negative health consequences in both the short and long term compared with women with no history of domestic violence. Disabling health problems for women survivors may persist for many years after the abuse has ended. Midwives can help women by understanding their situation, giving supportive messages and recognizing the potential adverse health consequences that an underlying history of domestic violence can have on the women for whom they are caring during pregnancy and labour, and after childbirth.

This chapter makes the connection between domestic violence and health promotion. It explores some of the health promotion strategies that midwives can use in their daily practices, in order to make a significant difference to the health of women and their babies during the childbearing years. The evidence that has shown that domestic violence is a threat to public health and the health of women before and during pregnancy and after childbirth is reviewed. The chapter draws on research that has explored inter-ventions for domestic violence in maternity and primary care settings, and identifies the implications for the role of the midwife in health promotion. In conclusion, the importance of midwives working collaboratively and in partnership with statutory and front-line workers from specialist domestic violence agencies is highlighted. Terms such as 'abused woman', 'violence against women' and 'intimate partner violence' are used interchangeably with 'domestic violence' on purely grammatical and pragmatic grounds. These are all terms that have been used by health professionals, researchers and seminal writers both inside and outside the United Kingdom.

OVERVIEW AND EPIDEMIOLOGY OF DOMESTIC VIOLENCE

Although domestic violence is now recognized by national and international bodies as one of the most pervasive and pernicious forms of violence against women, there is no single, agreed definition of domestic violence or any agreed single definition of violence against women (British Council 1999, Macdonald 2002, Kelly and Lovett 2005). That said, most definitions include behaviours such as physical violence, sexual assaults, threats and psychological abuse. Studies have found that physical violence in intimate relationships is almost always accompanied by psychological abuse and this happens in a third to over a half of cases of sexual abuse (British Council 1999). For the purposes of this chapter domestic violence has been defined as:

> Any violence between current or former partners in an intimate relationship, wherever and whenever the violence occurs. The violence may include physical, sexual, emotional or financial abuse.
>
> Walby and Allen (2004, p. 4)

The above definition includes domestic violence by both current and former partners regardless of the legal or domiciliary status of the relationship. Although women can be violent towards men in relationships, and violence exists in homosexual, bisexual, transgender and lesbian partnerships, there is remarkable consistency across the evidence that it is predominately women in an intimate partner relationship who are most at risk of suffering domestic violence (World Health Organization (WHO) 2002, Home Office 2003). Statistics on domestic violence are of three kinds:

1. Incidence: the number of new cases in a given time period (often 1 year).
2. Prevalence: the proportion of a population who have ever experienced domestic violence (therefore rates are always higher than those for incidence).
3. Reported cases: those known to and recorded by agencies, usually over an annual time-frame (Kelly 1998).

Unlike many other industrialized countries, there is no national British prevalence study of domestic violence. Surveys conducted elsewhere suggest a lifetime prevalence of domestic violence against women at between 25 and 30 per cent, with an annual prevalence rate of between 2 and 12 per cent. Variability in these estimates has been attributed in part to differences in the definitions used in the survey, e.g. whether emotional and verbal abuse, stalking and rape had been included (WHO 2002). Despite these caveats to uncovering the prevalence of domestic violence, research that ranges from large-scale surveys to participatory research has resulted in a widespread understanding of the scale of the problem. One of the most detailed and rigorous surveys to date was completed by Statistics Canada in the early 1990s (Johnson 1996). The Canadian survey supports the findings of a variety of studies worldwide, including the UK, e.g. in Canada's 1993 national violence survey one in four women had experienced domestic violence from their partner or ex-partner, and a third of women who were abused physically in a relationship said that they had feared for their lives at some point in time. These figures are remarkably consistent with those in the UK, where one in four women experiences some form of violence in their lifetime and every week two women die as a result of it (Home Office 2003). Apart from the individual human costs incurred by domestic violence, the economic impact and costs to society should not be underestimated. A recent study estimated that the total cost of intimate partner violence in the UK to victims, employers and the state was in the region of £23 billion (Walby 2004).

An important and illuminating source of information for midwives on domestic violence in the UK comes from the London Metropolitan Police Service (2001a). During the first 6 months of 2001, there were 44 476 allegations of domestic violence recorded by the Metropolitan Police Service. This is equivalent to one contact every 6 minutes. An in-depth analysis of a day count of all allegations recorded by the police revealed the following:

- More than 1 in 20 incidents involved a woman who was pregnant, and in several other cases the woman had recently given birth.
- More than 1 in 8 cases recorded issues around child contact or disputes over custody.
- In more than 1 in 15 incidents the perpetrator made use of an object or a weapon to threaten and/or hurt the victim.
- The types of injuries sustained included bite marks, bruising, cuts, split lips, and puncture, slash and stab wounds.
- Many of the victims reported that they were shocked, distressed and/or afraid.
- Property was damaged in 1 in 12 cases.

These findings highlight that women of childbearing age are at particular risk of experiencing domestic violence, and its impact on women and their children is profound. Moreover, the above findings need to be considered in the context of the studies that have shown that many incidences of domestic violence go unreported, and that victims of domestic violence are more likely to become repeat victims than for any other type of crime. Domestic violence is also more likely to result in injury than other types of assault. In comparison to other types of assault, those subjected to domestic violence are more likely to be upset and frightened by the incident, in both the short and the long term (Metropolitan Police Service 2001a). The effects of domestic violence on women's health and mental well-being are substantial and are discussed in more detail below.

PHYSICAL HEALTH EFFECTS OF DOMESTIC VIOLENCE

Domestic violence compromises the physical health of women and can result in poor health status, high use of health services, poor quality of life and adverse pregnancy outcomes (Campbell 2002, Keeling and Birch 2004). Risk behaviours such as smoking and substance abuse have been shown to be coping strategies for some women in abusive relationships (Grimstad et al. 1998). Although it can be difficult to isolate causal pathways to account for the effects of domestic violence, there is no doubt that injuries to the bodies of women as a direct result of domestic violence are very common. A wide range of studies has shown that bruising on the body is one of the most common injuries sustained by pregnant and non-pregnant women during violent events (Dobash et al. 1996, Aston 2003). The literature documents that injuries and bruising are often located in the head, face, neck, thorax, breasts, shoulders, back and abdomen (Stewart and Cecutti 1993, Dobash et al. 1996, Aston 2003). These findings suggest that, during the physical examinations of women during pregnancy and labour, and after delivery, midwives need to keep these body sites in mind as potential markers of physical abuse. The current evidence suggests that midwives and all maternity care professionals who work in the field need to be cognisant not only of the morbidity associated with intimate partner violence but also of the numbers of women whose lives are threatened and at risk as a result of domestic violence. The Metropolitan Police Service reviewed the cases of 56 women murdered by a partner in London between 2001 and 2002, and sexual assault and pregnancy/new births were identified as two of the six risk factors for homicide. Here it is important to note that in the murder review it states that 'victims who are assaulted whilst pregnant or when they have just given birth should be considered as high risk. This is in terms of future harm to them and to the child' (Richards 2003, p. 37).

Apart from the unnecessary suffering, distress or even death caused by direct injuries, domestic violence can result in women experiencing other physical health problems, which have been reported by Chamberlain (2004) and Campbell (2002) (Box 14.1). Midwives are recommended to bear in mind that, if women have suboptimal weight gain during pregnancy, this may be associated with women's experiences of domestic violence.

DOMESTIC VIOLENCE AND WOMEN'S SEXUAL HEALTH

To promote the health of women experiencing sexual violence during and after pregnancy, midwives need to be aware of the links between domestic violence and

---

Box 14.1 Physical health problems associated with intimate partner violence

- Headaches
- Recurring central nervous system symptoms including fits
- Migraines
- Back pain
- Cardiac symptoms such as hypertension and chest pain
- Gastrointestinal symptoms and problems, e.g. irritable bowel syndrome, eating disorders, poor appetite and weight loss

sexual assault. Sexual violence crosses the domains of women's health, sexuality and childbearing, and research on domestic violence and the abuse of women has capitalized on this overlap. Studies have shown that a substantial proportion of women experiencing physical violence also experience sexual violence, and it can have devastating sexual, medical, emotional and mental health consequences (Nehls and Sallmann 2005). Across these studies, it seems that most women endure vaginal and/or anal penetration and direct physical force. Rape-related pregnancy rates of between 4 and 5 per cent per rape each year have been identified (Holmes et al. 1996, Walby and Allen 2004). Women with unintended pregnancies are at increased risk of physical abuse around the time of pregnancy compared with women whose pregnancies are intended (Campbell et al. 1995).

A seminal study by Campbell and Alford (1989) of women living in battered women's shelters found that over 80 per cent of women respondents reported vaginal rape, over 50 per cent reported anal rape and just under 30 per cent reported objects being forcefully put into the vagina or anus. In addition, 44 per cent reported being hit, kicked or burned during sex. Campbell and Alford also found that women were often threatened with a beating or actually beaten after refusing sex. And, finally, a key finding with obvious implications for midwives and their practice was that nearly 50 per cent of women reported being coerced into having sex after hospital discharge and this was most often after childbirth.

Midwives are in the unique position to care for the sexual health of women during pregnancy, childbirth and early family beginnings (Aston 2005). Thus, midwives need to be aware, first, of the context of sexual violence against women and, second, of the serious health problems that can result as a consequence of the heinous crime of sexual abuse of women. The London Metropolitan Police Service (2001b) recently conducted a detailed analysis of 175 domestic sexual assault incidents and the findings included the following:

- Six victims were pregnant at the time of the assault.
- One in two partners was separated or separating at the time of the offence.
- Children were present during the assault in one in four situations.
- Three in four victims had made previous reports of domestic violence to the police.
- One in four victims wanted to pursue the allegation.
- Three in four victims did not want to pursue, citing: concern for children; fear of not being believed; vulnerability; fear of retaliation; and fear of the court process.

These findings highlight the seriousness of sexual violence, in terms not only of prevalence during pregnancy but also of the multiple victimizations of women. In addition they show some of the forms that children's contact with and experiences of violence towards their mother can take. Pregnancy and gynaecological complications have consistently been found to be related to sexual violence, including (Campbell 2002, WHO 2002):

- multiple hospitalizations during pregnancy
- genital and non-genital injuries
- sexually transmitted infections including HIV
- vaginal bleeding or infection
- decreased libido
- genital irritation
- dyspareunia

> ## Box 14.2   Strategies and practices that midwives can use to help women talk about the violence in their lives
>
> - Create an environment that is safe and private for assessment and disclosure
> - During appointments with women arrange to have some time with them by themselves without their partners
> - Never use partners or relatives to act as interpreters
> - Believe women who disclose abuse and offer supportive messages
> - Recognize the impact of sexual violence on women's health
> - Provide information and educate women about ways of keeping themselves safe
> - Provide information and educate women about their options regarding safety
> - Give women information about local service provision, community resources, and statutory and voluntary agencies
> - Liaise with and refer to other health professionals and relevant agencies as appropriate while taking account of the individual needs and wishes of women

- chronic pelvic pain
- urinary tract infections.

Moreover, research on the effect of intimate partner violence on reproductive decision-making has shown that women are often fearful of raising the issue of contraception or condom use. In sum, the current evidence suggests that domestic violence and sexual violence against women during their childbearing years appear to feed off each other and each form appears to predispose to the other. Sexual violence usually includes the use of physical force to compel a woman to engage in a sexual act against her will.

Sexual violence against women is not a rare event and it has serious consequences for women's health. Box 14.2 shows some health-promoting strategies and practices that midwives can use in order to help women talk about the violence in their lives.

DOMESTIC VIOLENCE DURING PREGNANCY

Research on domestic violence during pregnancy has focused primarily on the prevalence of the problem. Comparing results between studies can be difficult because dissimilar screening instruments, study populations, settings and non-standardized definitions of domestic violence have been used. Higher prevalence rates appear to be associated with more inclusive definitions of domestic violence, direct questioning by trained health professionals and repeated questioning (Bacchus et al. 2001). Studies examining the prevalence of domestic violence during pregnancy have noted ranges between 0.9 and 33.7 per cent of pregnant women, but in most studies prevalence rates of between 3 and 8 per cent have been reported (Gazmararian et al. 1996, Bacchus et al. 2004). Midwives need to be aware of the growing body of research that reveals that intimate partner violence among adolescents is more prevalent than previously assumed. Research has shown that adolescents and young women represent a significant proportion of the individuals affected by abuse during pregnancy. In some studies prevalence rates of domestic violence that are higher than those for pregnant adult women have been reported (Harrykissoon et al. 2002).

Midwives should never underestimate the risks to young women under the age of 18 years. This is highlighted in the findings of the latest *Why Mothers Die* report where 62 per cent of the deaths of schoolgirls or young women under the age of 18 years had suffered violence in the home (Lewis and Drife 2004). In sum, what the vast majority of all the prevalence studies show is that domestic violence is a common occurrence during pregnancy and there is reason to believe it may be more common than conditions such as diabetes and pre-eclampsia, for which women are routinely screened in pregnancy (Bacchus et al. 2001). Some studies have suggested that domestic violence can start or escalate during pregnancy, or that pregnancy can be associated with a reduction in violence (Bacchus et al. 2001). During pregnancy women experiencing domestic violence are thought to be more likely to sustain an injury to the abdomen, breasts and genital area (Bacchus et al. 2001). Moreover, the risk of domestic violence during pregnancy appears to be increased if women experience it before pregnancy (Bacchus et al. 2003).

Health consequences of domestic violence during pregnancy

The main health effects of domestic violence during pregnancy are the threat to health and the risk of death of the mother, fetus or both from trauma (Campbell 2002). Many studies have noted associations of abuse during pregnancy with adverse maternal and infant outcomes such as: miscarriage; low birthweight; pre-term labour and delivery; fetal distress; fetal injury or death; placental separation and antepartum haemorrhage; and rupture of the uterus, liver or spleen (Chamberlain 2004, El Kady et al. 2005). Other documented outcomes associated with domestic violence in pregnancy have included increased risk of miscarriage, stillbirth and chorioamnionitis (Campbell 2001). These studies have documented the outcomes that can compromise the health of women and their unborn babies. Midwives already make a substantial contribution to the social and public health aspects of maternity care and play a key role in providing health education. Thus, they are ideally placed to offer early access to services and interventions to women experiencing domestic violence. However, it is recognized that women experiencing domestic violence are more likely to be socially isolated, book late or be poor or non-attenders at antenatal care clinics. The role of the midwife is to ensure that any barriers to accessing maternity services are recognized and removed (Aston 2004).

It is now recognized that the risks associated with domestic violence can be acute and life threatening. Women who experience domestic violence during pregnancy have been identified as at increased risk of physical and emotional problems, and for maternal homicide (Richards 2003). In the findings of the latest *Why Mothers Die* report, 12 women had been murdered by their partner during or shortly after pregnancy (Lewis and Drife 2004). Another 43 women whose deaths were reported to the Enquiry had either voluntarily reported violence to a health-care professional during their pregnancy or were already known to be in an abusive relationship. The 55 women who died represent 14 per cent of the 391 women whose deaths were reported to the latest Enquiry. None of the women had been routinely asked about violence as part of their social history, and as a result the Enquiry concluded that 14 per cent was probably an underestimate. Although a full account of the findings and recommendations of the Enquiry are beyond the scope of this chapter, the implications for the role of the midwife are clearly and unequivocally set out in the report of the Enquiry. Midwives have a professional responsibility and accountability to familiarize themselves with the findings and the recommendations, and then to act accordingly. Midwives need to be constantly vigilant and alert for possible risk factors and signs of domestic violence during pregnancy. The reality is that the violence against women during pregnancy places women in danger and is sometimes lethal.

DOMESTIC VIOLENCE AFTER CHILDBIRTH

Studies have found that for some women domestic violence gets worse after the birth of their babies (Gielen et al. 1994, Mezey and Bewley 1997, Aston 2003). Research has indicated that women experience a significant increase in the mean number of incidents of moderate or severe physical abuse at 3 and 6 months, respectively, after childbirth, when compared with the incidents of violence that they experienced during pregnancy, e.g. Gielen et al. (1994) found that 19 per cent of their sample reported experiencing moderate or severe physical abuse during pregnancy, whereas 25 per cent reported moderate or severe violence in the postpartum period. Although another study did not find an increase in the prevalence of physical abuse after pregnancy, 6.1 per cent during pregnancy and 3.2 per cent during a mean postpartum period of 3.6 months, the study found that 77 per cent of the women who were abused after pregnancy were injured, but only 23 per cent received medical treatment for their injuries (Martin et al. 2001).

Other studies have indicated that younger mothers are at greater risk of physical violence after the birth of their babies than during pregnancy (Harrykissoon et al. 2002). In the first prospective study to examine the prevalence of physical violence among adolescent girls, aged 18 years and younger, who gave birth over a 2-year time span, the overall rate of violence during the 24-month postpartum period was 41 per cent. The highest (21 per cent) prevalence of physical violence occurred during the first 3 months after childbirth and lowest at 24 months post partum (13 per cent). Although the overall prevalence decreased over the study period, the proportion defined as severe physical violence increased from 40 per cent to 63 per cent by 24 months. In this study three of four adolescents reporting violence 3 months after delivery did not report violence during pregnancy (Harrykissoon et al. 2002).

The evidence in these studies and others suggests that midwives are frequently and sometimes unknowingly in contact with abused women after childbirth. Although midwives have reported examining women with torn perineal sutures attributed to forced vaginal penetration after childbirth, there is evidence to suggest that domestic violence can either be unrecognized by midwives or not be disclosed by the women (Hunt and Martin 2001). Aston (2003) found that living with domestic violence and coping with the demands of a new baby were a significant source of women's emotional and psychological distress. Aston also reported that women in her study were preoccupied with concerns about the safety of their babies during violent events because they could occur when women were involved in the care and feeding of their babies. Clearly, it is incumbent on midwives to support women so they do not feel that they have to cope alone with the abuse in order to achieve a measure of safety for themselves and their babies. Box 14.3 gives some health-promoting strategies and practices that midwives can use to support women.

Box 14.3   Health-promoting strategies and practices that midwives can use to support women

- Be aware that domestic violence may begin or get worse after childbirth
- Listen to what women are telling you and always believe them if they disclose abuse
- During physical examinations of women be alert for signs of injuries (they may be hidden)
- Ask women about domestic violence in private during postnatal visits
- Be alert to the connection between postnatal depression and domestic violence
- Identify the sources of support that women use
- Offer women more frequent home visits
- Build upon women's coping strategies
- Be alert to the research that has identified domestic violence as a risk factor for child abuse
- Follow national and local policies and guidelines on multi-agency child protection services

Please refer to the previous box because many of the strategies and practices that are included are relevant at this point and not repeated here.

DOMESTIC VIOLENCE AND WOMEN'S MENTAL HEALTH

Women with a history of domestic violence are more likely to experience some mental health issues (Mezey et al. 2005). Physical, sexual and psychological abuses by an intimate partner have all been associated with significant mental health difficulties in women (Women's Aid 2005). These include depression, anxiety, sleep problems, eating disorders, post-traumatic stress disorder, self-harming behaviour and suicide ideation/actions. Women's Aid (2005, p. 1) reported that 'these might result from the abuse, or predate it; experience of abuse can also exacerbate an existing condition. Sometimes these problems are very severe, and require inter-vention from mental health professionals'. The research evidence suggests that between 50 and 60 per cent of women who access mental health services have experienced domestic violence, and up to 20 per cent will be experiencing current abuse (Women's Aid 2005). In recent studies domestic violence and other abuse have been found to be the most prevalent cause of depression and other mental health difficulties in women.

If midwives are to promote health and address the psychological and mental health needs of women, they need to identify women who have a history of domestic violence or are currently experiencing violence. To work most effectively with women and address their psychological needs midwives need to:

- provide individualized woman-centred care (Aston 2004)
- recognize the combined stressors that coping with the demands of a new baby, domestic violence and mental distress can bring
- optimize midwifery care by providing women with extra support
- seek out and make links with appropriate perinatal and mental health services.

'ROUTINE ENQUIRY', 'SCREENING' AND ASKING ABOUT DOMESTIC VIOLENCE IN MATERNITY CARE SETTINGS

The terms in the title of this section have all been used at some time to describe the ways in which maternity and other health professionals may be able to identify women who are at risk of, or have already experienced, domestic violence. For an analysis of some of the debates around the use of the term 'screening' for domestic violence in pregnancy, see Bacchus and Aston (2005). Against a background of contested views and attention-grabbing newspaper headlines regarding pregnant women and domestic violence, which have been played out recently in the broadsheet and tabloid press, the current policy agenda focuses on the use of routine enquiry about domestic violence as part of the social history at the booking visit or at another opportune moment during the antenatal period (Lewis and Drife 2004). Routine enquiry has been defined as involving 'asking about the experience of domestic violence of all people within certain parameters' (DoH 2000, p. 23), regardless of visible signs of abuse, or whether domestic violence is suspected (Hester and Westmarland 2005). Routine enquiry has the advantage of not stigmatizing women. Studies conducted in maternity settings in the USA have found that selective screening based on a maternity care professional's perception of risk meant that incorrect judgements and negative assumptions were made about 'only certain types' of women who experience domestic violence (Clark et al. 2000).

Reflection – 1

Have you got any ideas about which 'types' of women were thought to be more at risk for experiencing domestic violence? Write these ideas down and consider them again after reading this chapter.

Routine enquiry gives women the opportunity to disclose their experiences of domestic violence and it provides midwives with the opportunity to ensure that women receive a sympathetic and non-judgemental hearing, information about specialized domestic violence support services and safety planning (Bacchus et al. 2001, Taket 2004, McVeigh et al. 2005). Systematic reviews on screening for domestic violence in health-care settings have reported that screening is acceptable to most women but that acceptance among health professionals in hospital and primary care settings is somewhat lower (Hester and Westmarland 2005). Domestic violence is a sensitive issue and talking about it during professional consultations can be difficult.

Individual practitioners may find that domestic violence raises uncomfortable and painful personal questions and experiences of violence and abusive relationships in their own lives. In addition, clinicians have reported that lack of knowledge and adequate training, lack of time, the inability to obtain confidential and one-to-one time with women and fear of opening a 'Pandora's box' are barriers to enquiring about domestic violence in maternity and other health-care settings (Bacchus et al. 2003). Higher rates of disclosure of domestic violence have been observed in response to direct questioning by trained health professionals and repeated questioning (Bacchus et al. 2001). Training is required on routine enquiry for domestic violence because midwives need to learn, first, how to identify abuse, second, how to question women safely and sensitively, third, how to respond appropriately to disclosure of abuse and, finally, they need to be familiar with national and local policies and guidelines on domestic violence and the services and agencies to which women can be referred (Salmon et al. 2004).

Activity – 1

How can personal biases and negative assumptions about women who experience domestic violence be challenged and addressed?

MIDWIVES WORKING IN PARTNERSHIP

Domestic violence is a threat to the lives and health of women and no community remains untouched by it. Over the last two decades much has been achieved to reform and strengthen the laws, policies, practices and responses to domestic violence across the criminal justice, and health and social care systems. The driving force for many of these changes has been organizations and charities such as the Women's Aid Federation of England and Refuge. For 30 years Women's Aid has campaigned to protect abused women and children. They work closely with the Government and many different national and local agencies and services, and are recognized as the experts on domestic violence (Women's Aid 2004).

The Government believes that no one organization can address domestic violence in isolation and the National Health Science has an important contribution to make in improving effective, integrated and early preventive responses for survivors of domestic violence. One of the challenges to partnership working on domestic violence is the need for guidance on the exchange of information between agencies. To aid closer partnership working the authors of a recently published report have called for greater clarity and 'clear national guidance on the exchange of information related to violence, especially between health and judicial systems. Such guidance should cover both anonymized and identifiable information' (McVeigh et al. 2005, p. 126). The role of the midwife is to promote joint working between agencies that supports women and not to try to 'fix' domestic violence or to tell women what to do (Chamberlain 2004). Midwives are uniquely situated to provide women with culturally appropriate care and to work collaboratively across sectors and in partnerships in order to promote safe coordinated responses to domestic violence.

SUMMARY OF KEY POINTS

- Domestic violence can have devastating impacts on the physical, mental, sexual and reproductive health of women during their childbearing years.
- Midwives need to build upon what is known already and what has been accomplished to improve the health of women experiencing domestic violence.

- Midwives need education, training and support in order to enquire about and help prevent domestic violence during pregnancy.
- Midwives play a crucial role in establishing whether women are at risk or have experienced any domestic violence during pregnancy and after childbirth.
- Midwives can make a difference because they are in prime position to offer women experiencing domestic violence individualized early interventions, support and advice.
- Partners or relatives should not be used to act as translators and the use of professional female interpreters is imperative.
- Midwives will need support and guidance from management and professional organizations to deal with, and respond to, the sensitive area of the overlap between domestic violence and the abuse of infants and children.
- Up-to-date written information about domestic violence should be displayed and available for women to read and take away in maternity, primary and sexual health services.
- Midwives need to promote primary and secondary prevention responses to domestic violence.
- It is recognized that there is a need for more research on domestic violence prevention, and the effectiveness and consequences of interventions in maternity and health-care settings.

REFERENCES

Aston G (2003) From the margins into the centre: women's experiences of domestic violence during pregnancy. Unpublished PhD thesis, University of Manchester.

Aston G (2004) The silence of domestic violence in pregnancy during women's encounters with maternity and healthcare professionals. *RCM Midwives* **7**: 165–6.

Aston G (2005) Sexuality during and after pregnancy. In: Andrews G (ed.), *Women's Sexual Health*, 3rd edn. London: Elsevier Ltd, pp. 169–97.

Bacchus L, Aston G (2005) 'To screen or not to screen: that is the question' … or is it? – asking about domestic violence during pregnancy. *NCT Journal New Digest* **31**: 8–9.

Bacchus L, Bewley S, Mezey G (2001) Domestic violence in pregnancy. *Fetal and Maternal Medicine Review* **12**: 249–71.

Bacchus L, Mezey G, Bewley S (2003) Experiences of seeking help from health professionals in a sample of women who experienced domestic violence. *Health and Social Care in the Community* **11**: 10–18.

Bacchus L, Mezey G, Bewley S, Haworth A (2004) Domestic violence: prevalence in pregnant women and associations with physical and psychological health. *European Journal of Obstetrics and Gynaecology and Reproductive Biology* **113**: 6–11.

British Council (1999) *Violence Against Women: A briefing document on international issues and responses.* Manchester: The British Council.

Campbell JC (2001) Abuse during pregnancy: a quintessential threat to maternal and child health – so when do we start to act? *Canadian Medical Association Journal* **164**: 1578–9.

Campbell JC (2002) Violence against women II: health consequences of intimate partner violence. *The Lancet* **359**: 1331–6.

Campbell JC, Alford P (1989) The dark consequences of marital rape. *American Journal of Nursing* **89**: 946–9.

Campbell JC, Pugh LC, Campbell D, Vissher M (1995) The influence of abuse on pregnancy intention. *Women's Health Issues* **5**: 214–23.

Chamberlain L (2004) *Making the Connection: Domestic violence and public health.* San Francisco, CA: The Family Violence Prevention Fund.

Clark KA, Martin SL, Petersen R et al. (2000) Who gets screened during pregnancy for partner violence? *Archives of Family Medicine* **9**: 1093–9.

Department of Health (2000) *Domestic Violence: A resource manual for health care professionals.* London: DoH.

Department of Health (2004) *Health Minister Announces New Steps to Aid Victims of Domestic Violence.* Press release reference number 2004/0376. London: DoH.

Dobash RP, Dobash RE, Cavanagh K, Lewis R (1996) *Research Evaluation of Programmes for Violent Men.* Edinburgh: The Scottish Office Central Research Unit.

El Kady D, Gilbert WM, Xing G, Smith LH (2005) Maternal and neonatal outcomes of assaults during pregnancy. *Obstetrics and Gynecology* **105**: 357–63.

Gazmararian JA, Lazorick S, Spitz AM, Ballard TJ, Saltzman LE, Marks JS (1996) Prevalence of violence against pregnant women. *Journal of the American Medical Association* **275**: 1915–20.

Gielen AC, O'Campo PJ, Faden RR, Kass NE, Xue X (1994) Interpersonal conflict and physical violence during the childbearing years. *Social Science and Medicine* **39**: 781–7.

Grimstad H, Backe B, Jacobsen G, Schei B (1998) Abuse history and health risk behaviours in pregnancy. *Acta Obstetrica et Gynecologica Scandinavica* **77**: 893–7.

Harrykissoon SD, Rickert VI, Weimann CM (2002) Prevalence and patterns of intimate partner violence among adolescent mothers during the postpartum period. *Archives of Pediatric and Adolescent Medicine* **156**: 325–30.

Hester M, Westmarland N (2005) *Tackling Domestic Violence: Effective interventions and approaches.* Home Office Research Study 290. London: Home Office Research, Development and Statistics Directorate.

Holmes MM, Resnick HS, Kilpatrick DG, Best CL (1996) Rape-related pregnancy: estimates and descriptive characteristics from a national sample of women. *American Journal of Obstetrics and Gynecology* **175**: 320–5.

Home Office (2003) *Safety and Justice: The Government's proposals on domestic violence.* London: The Stationery Office.

Hunt SC, Martin AM (2001) *Pregnant Women: Violent men – what midwives need to know.* Oxford: Books for Midwives.

Johnson H (1996) *Dangerous Domains: Violence against women in Canada.* Scarborough, Ontario: Nelson Canada.

Keeling J, Birch L (2004) Asking pregnant women about domestic abuse. *British Journal of Midwifery* **12**: 746–9.

Kelly L (1998) Domestic violence: A UK perspective. *The Network Newsletter: Violence Against Women.* Newsletter No. 15. Manchester: The British Council.

Kelly L, Lovett J (2005) *What a Waste: The case for an integrated violence against women strategy.* London: Women's National Commission/Department of Trade and Industry.

Lewis G, Drife D (2004) *Why Mothers Die 2000–2002. Confidential Enquiry into Maternal and Child Health:* London: RCOG Press.

Macdonald G (2002) Violence and health: the ultimate public health challenge. *Health Promotion International* **17**: 293–5.

McVeigh C, Hughes K, Bellis MA, Reed E, Ashton JR, Syed Q (2005) *Violent Britain: People, prevention and public health.* Liverpool: Centre for Public Health, Liverpool John Moores University.

Martin SL, Mackie L, Kupper LL, Buescher PA, Moracco KE (2001) Physical abuse of women before, during, and after pregnancy. *Journal of the American Medical Association Journal* **285**: 1581–4.

Mezey G, Bewley S (1997) Domestic violence and pregnancy: risk is greatest after delivery. *British Medical Journal* **314**: 1295.

Mezey G, Bacchus L, Bewley S (2005) Domestic violence, lifetime trauma and psychological health of childbearing women. *British Journal of Obstetrics and Gynaecology* **112**: 197–204.

Metropolitan Police Service (2001a) *Understanding and Responding to Hate Crime Factsheets: Domestic Violence.* London: Metropolitan Police Service.

Metropolitan Police Service (2001b) *Understanding and Responding to Hate Crime Factsheets: Sexual Assaults.* London: Metropolitan Police Service.

Nehls N, Sallmann J (2005) Women living with a history of physical and/or sexual abuse, substance use, and mental health problems. *Qualitative Health Research* **15**: 365–81.

Price S (2003) Domestic violence. In: Squire C (ed.), *The Social Context of Birth.* Abingdon, Oxon: Radcliffe Medical Press Ltd, pp. 107–20.

Price S, Baird K, Salmon D (2005) Asking the question: antenatal domestic violence. *The Practising Midwife* **8**: 21–5.

Richards L (2003) *Findings from the Multi-agency Domestic Violence Murder Reviews in London. Prepared for the ACPO homicide working group.* London: Metropolitan Police Service: www.met.police.uk/csu/pdfs/MurderreportACPO.pdf

Royal College of Midwives (1997) Domestic abuse in pregnancy. *Position Paper No. 19.* London: RCM.

Salmon D, Baird K, Price S, Murphy S (2004) *An evaluation of the Bristol pregnancy and domestic violence programme to promote the introduction of routine antenatal enquiry for domestic violence at North Bristol NHS Trust.* Bristol: University of the West of England.

Stewart DE, Cecutti A (1993) Physical abuse in pregnancy. *Canadian Medical Association Journal* **149**: 1257–63.

Taket A (2004) *Tackling Domestic Violence: The role of health professionals.* Home Office Development and Practice Report 32. London: Home Office Research, Development and Statistics Directorate.

Walby S (2004) *The Cost of Domestic Violence.* London: Women and Equality Unit/ Department of Trade and Industry.

Walby S, Allen J (2004) *Domestic Violence, Sexual Assault and Stalking: Findings from the British Crime Survey.* Home Office Research Study 276. London: Home Office Research, Development and Statistics Directorate.

Women's Aid (2004) *Celebrating 30 years of Women's Aid 1974–2004.* Bristol: Women's Aid Federation of England.

Women's Aid (2005) Principles of good practice for working with women experiencing domestic violence: guidance for mental health professionals: www.womensaid.org.uk/ campaignsandresearch/health per cent20and%20dv%20campaign/health%20intro.htm (accessed May 2005).

World Health Organization (2002) *World Report on Violence and Health.* Geneva: WHO.

FURTHER INFORMATION

Freephone 24 hour National Domestic Violence Helpline run in partnership between Women's Aid and Refuge: 0808 2000 247

Respect phoneline for perpetrators: 0845 122 8609

FURTHER READING

Campbell JC (ed.) (1998) *Empowering Survivors of Abuse: Health care for battered women and their children*. London: Sage Publications Ltd.

Dobash RE, Dobash RP (1979) *Violence Against Wives: A case against the patriarchy*. New York: The Free Press.

Williamson E (2000) *Domestic Violence and Health: The response of the medical profession*. Bristol: The Policy Press.

15 THE ROLE OF COMPLEMENTARY AND ALTERNATIVE MEDICINE IN HEALTH PROMOTION

PENNY CHARLES

Midwives have been found to be the group of health professionals to use complementary therapies the most in their practice. Women also use many different complementary therapies to self-help when not pregnant and during pre-conception, pregnancy, labour and the postnatal period, and also to help facilitate the health of their partners and families. Complementary therapies may be provided by a midwife, who is suitably qualified, or a complementary practitioner trained in her or his own speciality. This chapter explores the role of complementary and alternative medicine (CAM) in health promotion and what it is about the therapies that works for midwives and women (even though there are few scientifically researched studies). Holism is the philosophy of care used in CAM. The use of case studies explores holism, working in partnership with women and the role of mind–body medicine (psychoneuroimmunology), which are all elements of CAM. Lastly, integration of CAM is discussed and how this could help to provide positive health promotion in midwifery.

DEFINITIONS OF COMPLEMENTARY AND ALTERNATIVE MEDICINE

To explore the role of complementary and alternative medicine (CAM) in health promotion it is necessary first to define what CAM is. The World Health Organization (WHO) defines traditional medicine (which we in the West call CAM) as:

> Health practices, approaches, knowledge and beliefs incorporating plant, animal and mineral based medicines, spiritual therapies, manual techniques and exercises, applied singularly or in combination to treat, diagnose and prevent illnesses or maintain well-being.

WHO (2003, p. 1)

The term 'complementary and alternative medicine' has evolved from combining both complementary therapies and alternative medicine into one category of health care. Complementary therapies may be defined as therapies that are complementary to orthodox medicine. More recently the term 'integrated health care' has been used for CAM, because this best reflects how therapies are being combined with conventional care (Russo 2000).

DIFFERENT CATEGORIZATIONS OF CAM

Some forms of CAM originate from Eastern philosophies of care such as traditional Chinese medicine (TCM) and Indian Ayurvedic medicine. There may be the use of acupuncture, acupressure or shiatsu in TCM and both of these Eastern practices may include massage, herbs, advice on diet and lifestyle, and practices such as meditation and yoga. These practices can be seen to promote health by bringing the body back into balance. The advice discussed would provide health education for the client.

There are other complete systems of healing such as osteopathy, chiropractic, homoeopathy and naturopathy, which can be considered more Western in origin, but they may be able to diagnose and treat conditions detrimental to health and provide different forms of health promotion.

A myriad of healing techniques such as spiritual healing, aromatherapy, reflexology, imagery, visualization and different types of massage are considered to be therapeutic. Often, clients experience deep relaxation effects, which are healing in themselves. The relaxation of the physical body will have a knock-on effect on the mind and spirit. In CAM, this holistic aspect recognizes that, when one area is treated, it is not in isolation and will have effects on other areas.

Lastly, women may use self-help methods such as breathing and relaxation techniques and may buy homoeopathic remedies, herbs, flower remedies and essential oils over the counter. All the different forms of CAM involve the woman taking responsibility for her own health and effectively promoting her own health, often in a holistic fashion.

The list of complementary therapies that may be used by women is extensive but even this may not be exhaustive (Box 15.1).

Box 15.1   Different types of complementary therapies used by women

- Acupuncture
- Alexander technique
- Aromatherapy
- Ayurvedic medicine
- Baby massage
- Bach flower remedies
- Bowen technique
- Breathing
- Buteyko
- Chiropractic
- Craniosacral therapy
- Crystal healing
- Dietary supplements
- Dowsing
- Hair analysis
- Herbal medicine
- Homoeopathy
- Hydrotherapy
- Hypnotherapy
- Imagery
- Iridology
- Kinesiology
- Massage
- Meditation
- Music
- Naturopathy
- Nutritional medicine
- Osteopathy
- Radionics
- Reflexology/reflex zone therapy
- Reiki
- Relaxation techniques
- Shiatsu
- Spiritual healing
- Tai Chi
- Therapeutic touch
- Traditional Chinese medicine
- Visualization
- Yoga

Tiran and Mack (2000, pp. 296–303) also list 'a chart for possible uses of complementary therapies for mother and baby' that is comprehensive and suggests what therapies can help with which condition.

Considering the increased usage of CAM, it is important as a health-care professional to be aware of how CAM has and is being assessed as efficacious and safe.

USE OF CAM IN MATERNITY CARE

The Government report on the use of CAM (House of Lords Select Committee on Science and Technology 2000) was instigated as a result of CAM becoming such a widely used form of health care. Coulter and Willis (2004) report on findings in 2000 in Australia of a 62 per cent increase in usage of CAM since 1993. They state that findings were similar for the UK. The National Institute for Clinical Excellence (NICE 2004) guidelines on antenatal care state that few complementary therapies have been established as safe and effective during pregnancy, so women should be advised to use them as little as possible in pregnancy. However, midwives are the health professionals who use complementary therapies most in their work (Liburd 1999), mainly as dual practitioners, because of demands from women.

Research

The debate as to the appropriateness of scientific research in CAM studies is well documented (Richardson 2000). The scientific approach regards randomized controlled trials as the gold standard for assessing efficacy. However, in CAM it is often difficult to reach any firm conclusions as a result of many factors. These may be caused by the differences in each individual being treated, the method and duration of treatment needed for the individual, the outcome measurement employed and the control intervention used. It is very difficult to know if positive results in the research process are the result of the effects of the therapy, the practitioner–client therapeutic relationship or other possibilities such as a placebo effect (this may be explained as the clients' expectations having an effect on the treatment outcome). However, Lewith et al. (2002) found that clients' expectations did not affect the clients' condition, thereby disputing this placebo assumption. It must also be recognized that, when scientific research has produced statistically significant results, those in traditional medicine may not take these on board. This may be because there are no explanations that satisfy orthodox science (at present) as to how some of these CAM methods work (as in the case of homoeopathy and spiritual healing).

There are numerous qualitative research studies and accounts from women reported in complementary therapy textbooks and journals, that show evidence of how these therapies can facilitate normal childbearing. Often women report feeling empowered by using CAM (Tiran 2004a) and midwives have reported feeling in touch with normal childbirth when using it (Yates 2003).

Activity – 1

Think what resources you could use to find out about complementary therapies, so that you are safe in your practice and so that you can help with giving informed choice to women.

(See suggestions in Box 15.2)

> ### Box 15.2 Methods for familiarizing yourself with complementary therapies
>
> - Treat yourself to a massage or a therapy with which you are unfamiliar
> - Ask lots of relevant questions (if you need to)
> - Reflect on the experience so that you may understand how and why it may be a health-promoting experience for women and families in your care
> - Find out if there are any midwives practising complementary therapies in your trust and work with them for a day or visit other units to see what is happening
> - Join the complementary therapy forum for health professionals
> - Go on a complementary therapy study day
>
> The Nursing and Midwifery Council (NMC) have produced the NMC's viewpoint as a position statement on the use of complementary and alternative therapies (NMC 2004) and midwives should be up to date with the Midwives Rules and Standards and the Code of Professional Conduct (NMC 2004) if they wish to use CAM in their practice, or even if they want to be able to give the women in their care informed choice. The importance is laid on being suitably qualified in the CAM, communicating with the members of the health team so that they are aware of the use of CAM therapy and gaining informed consent from the woman before using any forms of CAM.

HEALTH PROMOTION AND ITS RELATIONSHIP WITH CAM

Complementary and alternative medicine practitioners may see health promotion as being implicit within the therapies used. Women visit complementary therapists in order to stay well, to help facilitate a normal birth and to cope successfully with the addition of a new member of the family. The role of CAM in health promotion includes holism, a philosophy of care, which means that CAM practitioners work in partnership with women, facilitating empowerment.

Holism

One of the main reasons cited for why women use CAM is the use of holistic practice. The aim of holistic practice is to 'make whole', by helping the body heal itself or maintain a balance and therefore understanding the connection between the physical, mental, emotional and spiritual levels. Gaining information about the client is essential and includes a detailed history of physical, emotional, spiritual, social and lifestyle information, with an emphasis on what is important for that particular woman at that particular time. The CAM practitioner may work on one or several levels depending on the therapy used, with the knowledge that this will positively affect the whole person. In terms of health promotion, for example, it is acknowledged that working on promoting mental health will promote general well-being as illustrated in the first case study. In the second case study, work on a spiritual level illustrates this holistic effect by positively facilitating the woman and baby.

At the start of a CAM consultation information needs to be gathered. This takes up time, which may be at a premium in midwifery care, e.g. when the midwife is working in a busy antenatal clinic, women who book are often allocated a time slot (the average being 20 minutes). This may mean that there is no time to explore some issues in the necessary detail so that the woman feels that she has been able to tell her 'story' and adequately express any concerns. When home bookings occur without such a strict time allocation, women may feel more valued and that their story has been listened to. Midwives work hard with their communication skills, often by the combination of gaining an instant rapport, checking out professional judgements and intuitive/gut reaction skills with difficult staff resourcing and time-keeping problems. However, midwives and women are often dissatisfied with this system of care (Sandall 2004). Women who visit CAM practitioners (outside the realm of midwifery) are not restricted to the same tight time schedule, although there are necessary boundaries in place. However, the CAM practitioner wants and often needs to hear the woman's story, as this gaining of holistic information is vital to the treatment process. To promote health the CAM practitioner will be working at maintaining well-being and preventing problems arising. Rose's case study illustrates how CAM and, in this case, aromatherapy were able to work with some physical and mental health issues that were presented by Rose.

Case study: Rose

Rose, a multigravida, attended nine aromatherapy sessions throughout her pregnancy. Rose was anxious about the birth of this baby as a result of difficulties with two previous births. Rose also experienced stress caused by the uncertainty surrounding her partner's employment and the addition of a large extension to their house, involving living with a lot of dust and debris!

Minor problems were treated with essential oils or a combination of oils and massage. For one session Rose arrived with a heavy cold and a chesty cough, which was a contraindication to aromatherapy treatment. However, she did have a consultation and was sent away with antiviral and bactericidal oils to use in her bath.

Rose had a history of asthma. On occasions she arrived with some slight breathlessness. Frankincense (*Boswellia thurifera*) essential oil was used in her massage to very good effect. Frankincense can help to slow and steady the breathing, thus calming anxiety (Battaglia 1995). After this treatment Rose did not need to use her inhaler for 48–72 hours, a very positive response for someone who usually used it daily.

Rose suffered from some slight hand and foot oedema later on in pregnancy and this was successfully treated with geranium essential oil (*Pelargonium graveolus*).

Rose remained well throughout her pregnancy and this may have been a result of various factors in the CAM encounters. One of the factors may have been the support and time that Rose received from her aromatherapist, with the opportunity to tell her story, which promoted her mental health. Rose seemed able to work seamlessly through her anxieties and concerns simply by sharing them with the CAM practitioner. Rose's mental health was continuously promoted in this way. Another factor was a result of having her physical health promoted through a massage, which could work on her physical ailments. The effect of the massage was to create deep relaxation for Rose, which would have worked at all levels and promoted holistic health. The essential oils were chosen to work on whatever areas needed attention at that moment. Often the oils worked synergistically on different levels at the same time, which further complemented the care for Rose.

In the last month of pregnancy Rose and her partner were taught some very simple massage moves on the hands and arms (which could be transferred to other parts of the body) and a massage oil was made up for use in labour, so that her partner could carry on supporting Rose and also be happily occupied with a useful job. The advice was to massage for approximately 15 minutes every hour (Keenan 2000) or as Rose requested.

Activity – 2

List the ways of promoting health that were illustrated in Rose's case study.
(See health promotion list in Box 15.3)

The role of touch

Rose took responsibility for promoting her own health by choosing regular aromatherapy massage. When asked why she had come for aromatherapy Rose replied that she loved massage and wanted to 'treat' herself. Rose was making sure that she balanced a busy working and family life with time for herself. Touch would have played a very positive role for Rose. Results on research into massage show how an individual's self-esteem may be increased simply with regular use of caring touch. This can provide necessary confirmation and affirmation (Nathan 1999), which positively affect the person's mental and emotional health. In the case of Rose she may not have been aware that by choosing massage she was not only treating herself to an enjoyable experience (important in itself) but also helping herself to feel more

---

Box 15.3   Health promotion activities

Prevention of physical problems

1.   Chest infection prevented or ameliorated as a result of provision of essential oils
2.   Reduction of the need for daily inhaler use
3.   Reduced discomfort of oedema

Prevention of mental health problems

4.   Listening to Rose's story before the massage
5.   Giving Rose time to talk over her concerns

General overall prevention of stress

6.   Stress release as a result of regular massage and relaxed atmosphere
7.   Possible prevention of distress of partner by teaching him massage moves before labour
8.   Taught strategies for helping to cope in labour, if needed

confident about the workings of her own body. Massage could promote positive belief in her own body, which enabled and empowered Rose to cope in labour. This may have been achieved by Rose letting go to the labour process because she was more confident that her body knew what to do and was capable of doing it.

Massage and the role of touch have been shown to be very powerful promoters of holistic health. Numerous research studies into touch have shown how it can effectively promote mental health for individuals (Field 2000). The research on premature babies involved gentle stroking and the results showed heightened responsiveness and enhanced weight gain. Massage very effectively reduces anxiety and proved beneficial for adolescents with attention deficit hyperactivity disorder, autism, bulimia and depression (Field 2000). Research by Keenan (2000), where massage was used as part of the care for women coping with the pain of normal labour, produced positive obstetric outcomes. The Sure-Start initiative is using the results of research, which have shown that teaching women to massage their babies can prevent postnatal depression (Russo 2000).

WORKING IN PARTNERSHIP WITH WOMEN

Another reason cited for why women choose to see a complementary therapist is that clients want equal partnership in their health care. Many midwives would argue that, as autonomous practitioners, who care for women, there is little room for the reductionist approach, which is often a criticism of the doctor–patient relationship (Davis-Floyd and St John 1998). This approach is criticized for defining the woman by any problem that she may have, be it a minor pregnancy disorder or a more serious complication. There may be a distinct feeling of hierarchy with the woman feeling intimidated and subjected to a patriarchal approach to care, which can be detrimental to health promotion. It may be this style of care that shows the woman that the people in authority have the information and all she needs to do is follow orders, leaving a woman feeling disempowered and without the necessary knowledge to exercise control and choice.

In the case of Rose, who was taking responsibility for her health but also actively working in partnership with her CAM practitioner, she came to the aromatherapy sessions with different concerns to air each time. One example of how her mental health was supported was with an enquiry into iron-rich foods. Rose had received the information that her haemoglobin levels were low. Unfortunately, midwifery-staffing levels were very poor and she had not been able to discuss this issue with her midwife who would normally have been the professional to deal with this concern. Consequently she was left feeling confused and anxious about the meaning of this test, whether she could actively change the levels herself or whether she had no choice but to take the iron supplements prescribed for her. Together the client and CAM practitioner explored the foods and drinks that would increase and decrease iron levels plus alternatives to conventional iron supplements. Rose facilitated her own health promotion by sharing her concerns and educating herself in partnership with a CAM practitioner, who had the time to explore her worries and considered this time and exploration part of the holistic process. Rose consequently gained confirmation of the knowledge that she already had about iron-rich foods, gained some new information and subsequently felt more in control of her own health. This health education would also benefit her family in the future.

After discussion and reflection Rose decided to take the prescribed iron supplements; however, she could now also choose which foods to include (and which to cut out) in her diet in order to maintain optimum health. Rose was informed where to find the necessary health information and how to keep up to date (in books, leaflets and on the internet).

THE THERAPEUTIC RELATIONSHIP

There are many factors of the CAM encounter, and of holistic midwifery practice, that contribute to the therapeutic relationship, which is a necessary element of care. This therapeutic relationship involves value and support with the aim of empowerment and enabling the woman simply 'to be' (Mitchell and Cormack 1998). One part of the process of 'being' was found in the compassion shown by the health-care practitioner. Rose evaluated the aromatherapy sessions positively saying that the aromatherapist 'managed my changing shape and massage positions with delicacy and above all kindness'. In the event Rose had a normal birth and did not have the time or need for any extra support from her partner because she had a supportive midwife whom she also described as 'very kind'. Rose evidently valued this element of care in both the midwife and the CAM practitioner. The compassion that she experienced promoted mental health by working on an unconditional and accepting type of care. This kindness and compassion gave no room for any judgement and allowed Rose truly to be herself, which was another way of positively reinforcing Rose's sense of self, and led to self-empowerment, which consequently may have contributed in enabling her to cope better with the childbearing process. The connection between the mind and the body is well known and often seen clearly in midwifery. The science of mind–body medicine or psychoneuroimmunology is well respected in CAM (Fenwick 2001) and includes spiritual health care.

Psychoneuroimmunology

Psychoneuroimmunology (PNI) is 'the study of the intricate interaction of consciousness (psycho) brain and central nervous system (neuro) and the body's defence against infection and abnormal cell division (immunology)' (Fenwick 2001). Studies have shown that a positive affective response to circumstances, loving supportive relationships, optimism for the future and learning how to cope with psychological stresses may all keep our immune system healthy.

There are cases where the midwife can be in a position to practise her skills and let the woman express freely anxieties, emotions and fears that may be all that is needed to promote normal childbearing. However, sometimes there is an unanswered situation when there is no obvious reason for delay in the birthing process. Several types of CAM may be utilized to promote health in this situation, which means bringing the body into balance and harmony. Some examples of this are reflexology, homoeopathy and spiritual healing. In spiritual healing it is recognized that there is something more mystical and spiritual that surrounds childbirth and adds to its meaning. Parapsychological studies over the last 50 years have shown that the mind is not just limited to the skull (Fenwick 2001).

In the case of Lily she had support from her midwives, partner and friends. Lily could discuss any anxieties with the professionals and felt that she had done everything she could think of to promote her own health.

> ## Case study: Lily
>
> Lily was 41 weeks' pregnant and had planned a home birth but as she was now overdue there was concern from the doctor and midwife caring for Lily. The necessary tests regarding the health of her baby and the function of the placenta were booked for the following day. Distance healing was undertaken and revealed the need to welcome the baby positively, like a positive affirmation. Talking to Lily confirmed that, although Lily was delighted to be pregnant, she had some concerns, which she had openly discussed with the midwives and her partner. There was no obvious need for her to talk to anyone or to do anything any differently. Lily practised the positive affirmation concentrating on welcoming her baby and feeling love. That night Lily's waters broke and she went into spontaneous labour. Her baby was born at home.

The healer worked with the aim of providing the best possible help for Lily from a spiritual perspective, which may have picked up on a problem at any level: physical, mental, emotional, etc. The healer's perspective was of promoting balance through distance healing. This meant acting on the information received about the baby. The practice of positive affirmation recognized the interconnectedness of baby to mother, promoting spiritual health, and achieving balance and a normal birth. Although there is no proof that the healing helped because Lily may have gone into spontaneous labour without this intervention, Lily found the healing helpful and relaxing. In addition she achieved her choice and goal of a home birth. Lily reported feeling so supported that she would not want to undergo any subsequent pregnancies without a healer caring for her in a complementary fashion to the midwife (Charles 2003). Lily had not been consciously or actively concerned about her pregnancy and had been able to talk openly throughout her pregnancy to supportive carers. However, the healing had picked up on an area that was subconscious to the woman and that needed a positive affirmation in order to achieve harmony and wholeness.

Many different forms of CAM may find areas of imbalance of which the client is not aware and therefore over which she has no conscious control. These forms of CAM often look at the body in a very different way to orthodox medicine and so may be difficult to explain within a medical reductionist framework.

The case of Lily highlights the spiritual area of health promotion, which illustrates a belief that we are all interconnected on some level. When we can truly be with a woman as a midwife and truly be with a client as a CAM practitioner, this has been shown to promote health positively. This entails believing that women's bodies can work as they are meant to and that, unless there is a mechanical problem, women can birth their babies normally. The focus that a midwife or CAM practitioner has on the woman is vitally important to promote health. In physical terms this may mean maintaining eye contact, tuning into the woman's needs, or using or not using touch as necessary. At a mental level this may mean not letting our thoughts run away with us by, for example, compiling a list of what to buy for tea tonight, but keeping our awareness open positively to the woman's birthing process. The intention of the practitioner in CAM would be to make whole (and this would be the same for the midwife practising holistically). Often this would explicitly mean being there for the woman, being her advocate, and the woman knowing that she can trust the midwife/CAM practitioner.

Midwives are trained to work holistically, considering the woman as a whole person and working together with her in partnership, although often working in a medicalized environment may prevent the achievement of the best possible care for women undergoing a normal pregnancy as a result of the power dynamics (Sandall 2004). This may depend on the system of care in place, such as continuity of care and carer and midwifery group practices where it is easier to explore women's choices and subsequent control issues for women (Department of Health 2004).

INTEGRATION OF CAM

In the past a woman may not have shared with her midwife or GP that she was also seeing a CAM therapist for fear of being misunderstood. The therapist, however, was often all too aware that the client had used conventional medicine and had turned to CAM as a last resort or an alternative in the search for a clearer understanding of the problem or issue. It is now not unusual for a CAM therapist to communicate with the GP, midwife or whichever health professional is more appropriate in order to provide the best care for the woman and be able to promote health care. This has probably come about as a result of a combination of factors, including training of health professionals in CAM, who then include their CAM expertise in conventional medicine. This does of course depend on the individual practitioner. CAM therapies are often in the media and clients may well ask their primary carer about the use of CAM. It has now become important for health professionals to be able to talk about CAM therapies with their clients in order to give them informed choice.

Tiran (2004b) points out the benefits for women of 'dual knowledge'. It may be preferable for women to see a therapist who is educated in both a CAM therapy and the science and art of midwifery rather than a CAM specialist who is unfamiliar with the process of childbirth.

In my own practice as a spiritual healer, aromatherapist and midwife, I would aim to work in an integrated way. I would expect the woman to inform her midwife that she was having healing and/or aromatherapy. If necessary I would see it as within my role to talk to the professionals involved in the woman's care in order to promote best health for my client (after gaining the woman's consent).

CONCLUSION

Complementary and alternative medicine therapies are being integrated into midwifery to help promote normal birth. The push for integrated health is coming from women and midwives and being supported by CAM practitioners. Two different forms of CAM have illustrated (in the cases of Rose and Lily) how the promotion of mental and spiritual health achieved holistic health and may have facilitated normal birth. The role of CAM therapies in health promotion has been specifically through the empowerment of women to be themselves with compassion and support. This has been achieved by working in partnership with the woman in a therapeutic way and has shown how control and choice can be achieved for women in childbearing through the use of CAM therapies.

SUMMARY OF KEY POINTS

- Women, midwives and CAM practitioners use CAM therapies in midwifery.
- It is important to understand the meaning of holism, because it is this philosophy of care that facilitates health promotion.
- It is important for midwives to be informed about CAM therapies in order to offer informed choices to women.
- CAM therapies can enable working in partnership with women in a therapeutic manner, which is empowering.
- Midwives can be dual trained, which means that CAM therapies can be offered on the National Health Service and therefore be available to all women.
- Women, midwives and CAM practitioners need to communicate freely and work as a team in order to achieve integration.

REFERENCES

Battaglia S (1995) *The Complete Guide to Aromatherapy*. Australia: The Perfect Potion Pty Ltd.

Charles P (2003) Spiritual healing: Is there a place for its use in midwifery? *MIDIRS Midwifery Digest* **13**: 270–4.

Coulter I, Willis E (2004) The rise and rise of CAM: a sociological perspective. *Medical Journal Australia* **180**: 587–9.

Davis-Floyd R, St John G (1998) *From Doctor to Healer. The transformative journey*. London: Rutgers University Press.

Department of Health (2004) *National Service Framework for Children, Young People and Maternity Services*. London: The Stationery Office.

Fenwick P (2001) Psychoneuroimmunology: The mind–brain connection. In: Peters D (ed.), *Understanding the Placebo Effect in Complementary Medicine*. London: Churchill Livingstone, pp. 215–26.

Field T (2000) *Touch Therapy*. London: Churchill Livingstone.

House of Lords Select Committee on Science and Technology (2000) *Complementary and Alternative Medicine*. London: The Stationery Office.

Keenan P (2000) Benefits of massage therapy and use of a doula during labor and childbirth. *Alternative Therapies* **6**: 66–74.

Lewith G, Hyland M, Shaw S (2002) Do attitudes toward and beliefs about Complementary Medicine affect treatment outcome? *American Journal of Public Health* **92**: 1604–6.

Liburd A (1999) The use of complementary therapies in midwifery in the UK. *Journal of Nurse-Midwifery* **44**: 325–9.

Mitchell A, Cormack M (1998) *The Therapeutic Relationship in Complementary Health Care*. London: Churchill Livingstone.

Nathan B (1999) *Touch and Emotion in Manual Therapy*. London: Churchill Livingstone.

National Institute for Clinical Excellence (2004) *Antenatal Care. Routine care for the healthy pregnant woman*. London: The Stationery Office.

Nursing and Midwifery Council (2004) *Position Statement on Complementary Therapies*: www.nmc-uk.org (accessed November 2004).

Richardson J (2000) The use of randomized controlled trials in complementary therapies: exploring the issues. *Journal of Advanced Nursing* **32**: 398–406.

Russo H (2000) *Integrated Healthcare: A guide to good practice*. London: The Foundation for Integrated Healthcare.

Sandall J (2004) Normal birth is a Public Health Issue. *MIDIRS Midwifery Digest* **14** (suppl 1): 54–8.

Tiran D (2004a) Breech presentation: increasing maternal choice. *Complementary Therapies in Nursing and Midwifery* **10**: 233–8.

Tiran D (2004b) *Nausea and Vomiting in Pregnancy. An integrated approach to care*. London: Churchill Livingstone.

Tiran D, Mack S (eds) (2000) *Complementary Therapies for Pregnancy and Childbirth*, 2nd edn. London: Baillière Tindall.

World Health Organization (2003) *WHO Traditional Medicine. Fact Sheet No. 134*: www.who.int/mediacentre/factsheets/fs123/en/print/html (accessed January 2005).

Yates S (2003) *Shiatsu for Midwives*. London: Books for Midwives, Elsevier Science Ltd.

FURTHER READING

Field T (2002) Violence and touch deprivation in adolescents. *Adolescence* **37**: 735–49.

Glover V, Onozawa K, Hodgkinson A (2002) Benefits of infant massage for mothers with postnatal depression. *Seminars in Neonatology* **7**: 495–500.

Habek D, Habeck JC, Jagust M (2003) Acupuncture conversion of fetal breech presentation. *Fetal Diagnosis and Therapy* **18**: 418–21.

Hill F (2003) Complementary and alternative medicine: the next generation of health promotion? *Health Promotion International* **18**: 265–272.

Lewith G, Jonas W, Walach H (2002) *Clinical Research in Complementary Therapies*. London: Churchill Livingstone.

Mantle F (2002) The role of alternative medicine in treating postnatal depression. *Complementary Therapies in Nursing and Midwifery* **8**: 197–203.

Mollart L (2003) Single-blind trial addressing the differential effects of two reflexology techniques versus rest, on ankle and foot oedema in late pregnancy. *Complementary Therapies in Nursing and Midwifery* **9**: 203–8.

Tiran D, Chummun H (2004) Complementary therapies to reduce physiological stress in pregnancy. *Complementary Therapies in Nursing and Midwifery* **10**: 162–7.

Tovey P, Easthope G, Adams J (eds) (2004) *The Mainstreaming of Complementary and Alternative Medicine*. London: Routledge.

Weier K, Beal M (2004) Complementary therapies as adjuncts in the treatment of postpartum depression. *Journal of Midwifery and Women's Health* **49**: 96–104.

WEBSITES

Department of Health's (DoH) *National Service Framework for Children, Young People and Maternity Services: Maternity care*: www.dh.gov.uk.

Nursing and Midwifery Council (NMC): www.nmc-uk.org.

Prince of Wales's Foundation for Integrated Health (FIH): www.fihealth.org.uk.

Research Council for Complementary Medicine (RCCM): www.rccm.org.uk.

INDEX

Page numbers in **bold** indicate figures and tables